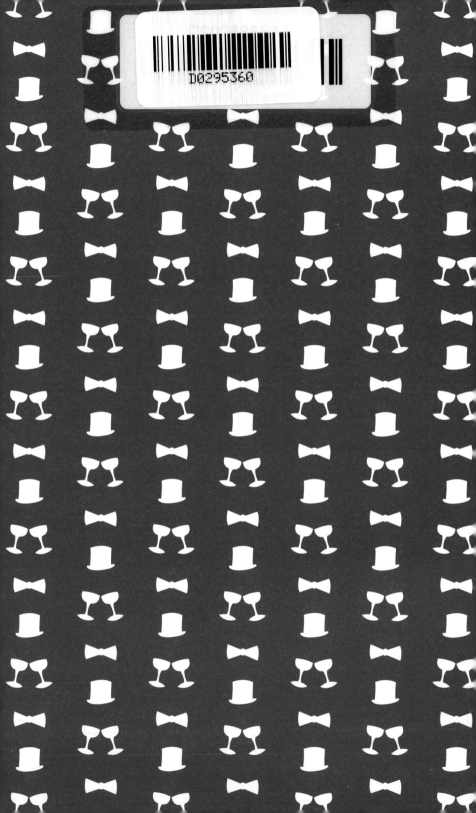

THREE MEN ON A DIET

Three Men on a Diet

*A Very English Approach
to Losing Weight*

GEORGE COURTAULD

CONSTABLE

CONSTABLE

Some names and details have been changed to protect the privacy of others.

First published in hardback in Great Britain in 2018 by Constable

1 3 5 7 9 10 8 6 4 2

Copyright © George Courtauld, 2018

The moral right of the author has been asserted.

A CIP catalogue record for this book
is available from the British Library.

ISBN: 978-1-47212-913-0

Typeset in Sabon by Hewer Text UK Ltd, Edinburgh
Printed and bound by CPI Group (UK) Ltd, Croydon, CR0 4YY

Papers used by Constable are from well-managed
forests and other responsible sources.

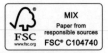

MIX
Paper from
responsible sources
FSC® C104740

Constable
An imprint of
Little, Brown Book Group
Carmelite House
50 Victoria Embankment
London EC4Y 0DZ

An Hachette UK Company
www.hachette.co.uk

www.littlebrown.co.uk

For my darling wife, Fiona, for her wisdom, beauty, forbearance – and cooking! With all my love.

CHAPTER 1

'Let your boat of life be light – one or two friends
worth the name, someone to love and someone to love
you, a cat, a dog and a pipe or two, enough to eat and
enough to wear, and a little more than enough to drink:
for thirst is a dangerous thing.'

Jerome K. Jerome, *Three Men in a Boat*

On almost the final working day before Christmas last year, I
pushed through the double front doors of the Spatchcock and
asked for Reggie Lambert.

'At the bar, sir,' the porter replied. 'He told me to send you
straight in.'

I hurried through the hall, past the large picture of a huge man
in Regency dress, affectionately known as Fat Jack, striding
doggedly down St James's, past the stairs and the grandfather
clock, to the bar, where the most senior and distinguished
member of the club, impossibly venerable, well dressed and
grand, was standing alone, staring with baffled hostility at an
empty tumbler. Of Reggie and the barman there was no sign.

He turned his grizzled aquiline head towards me and raised a pair of bushy eyebrows.

'Good morning,' he half bellowed. 'Looking for Reggie?'

'Yes,' I replied. 'I'm George Courtauld.' He grimaced in welcome but did not offer his hand.

'In the bog,' he snorted. 'Told me to get you a glass of champagne.' The barman appeared, thank goodness, now he had an ally, nodding and smiling. 'A glass of champagne on Mr Lambert's tab please, barman. ' The old man barked: 'And I'd better have another bullshot, please.' Then turning back to me, 'Are you the art dealer?'

'No, I'm a head-hunter.'

'*Really?*' He seemed strangely amazed. 'You look just like a banker.'

'The only people left who still do.'

'Yes. Yes. Now I come to think of it, you have a point. And where's your . . . your . . . *salon*, I suppose you call it?'

'My *office*,' I gently corrected him, 'is on Clifford Street, between Bond Street and Savile Row.'

'That must set you back a bob or two? But you're looking very well on it. How on earth did you get into that? I always assumed it was more of a . . . a ladies' game?'

'There are lots of very good women, naturally,' I replied, a touch defensively. 'But I think most of us are still men.'

'You do surprise me. And there's presumably some kind of formal training or apprenticeship? College or guild of some sort?'

'Well, it's completely unregulated, so one doesn't have to worry about official qualifications – or frankly any real training at all.'

2

'No wonder one sees so many shockers about. But you must have had some training?'

'No training, but a fair amount of relevant experience: I spent five years in the City, failing to make a bean for myself or anyone else, but I did make lots of friends who have been kind enough to push business my way ever since. I've been at it now for twenty-five years.'

'Good lord!' Watching the barman pass me a glass of champagne and begin mixing his bullshot, he softly jangled the change in his pockets.

'Now barman, I do apologise but I've forgotten your name: Completely senile of course. Is it Henry?'

'Yes, my lord,' Henry replied, draining his cocktail shaker into a fresh tumbler and passing it across to him.

'Thank you, Henry, thank you.' He took a restorative sip and raised his eyebrows at me again. 'I've often wondered, if you don't mind my asking, do you ever . . . do yourself?'

'Not yet,' I admitted. 'Very happy as I am.'

'I see. Imagined it must be rather difficult. But you're clearly quite exceptional, seriously top end. As we're talking shop, and the place is pretty much empty, perhaps you wouldn't mind telling me how much someone of your calibre . . . charges per job?'

'As much as I can possibly get away with; hopefully a minimum of . . . thirty thousand pounds . . .'

The old man coughed the bullshot straight back into his glass and sloshed it down his front.

'Thirty grand for a haircut?' he spluttered. 'No wonder you're looking so prosperous!' He whipped out a threadbare spotted

3

handkerchief and swabbed vigorously at his waistcoat. 'Well, you can certainly replace my bloody drink then.'

'I'm not a member, I'm afraid.' Only members were allowed to pay at the Spatchcock.

'No,' he answered drily. 'I suppose not. Where the hell is Reggie?'

'Here,' said a deep cheerful voice. 'Been chatting to Jane in trap two.' Mobile telephones, laptops, paperwork, receipts, business cards and female non-members of staff, among other things, are not allowed in the Spatchcock. To use a mobile telephone one has to go outside or shut oneself in a loo, as Reggie had been doing. 'She sends her love.'

'There you are, Reggie. Thought you were having triplets. Been talking to your hairdresser friend. Makes an absolute fortune.'

'He's a *head-hunter*. Not a hairdresser.'

'What?'

'A head-hunter. Are you going deaf?'

'Course not. Been deaf for years. Ha ha ha. Shooting.' He turned back to me. 'Head-hunter, eh? From Borneo?' Henry and I looked at each other. The old man slapped me on the back. 'Just joking. Must have misheard you. I know all about head-hunters.' He adopted a silly voice. '"Executive Search", don't they call it? Chilling. Ha ha ha. You had me going there for a minute.'

'Can I get you another drink?' Reggie offered.

'Do you know what, I think I'm off, thank you, Reggie. So sorry I can't help with Johnny Pinion, but he is now chairman after all. If people don't like him why on earth was he selected? Everyone keeps telling me what a terrible snob he is, but I rather like snobs.' He drained what was left of his drink and set the glass down on the bar. 'They're so terribly fond of me.' He threw his sodden handkerchief in the waste-paper basket. 'And anyway, isn't he supposed to be some sort of business guru or something? Language schools, isn't it? Communication, that's the key nowadays, or so I'm told. Might have some bright ideas. It's just not my place to lecture a chairman on how to behave in his own club. Pity, of course, but there it is.' He took three salted almonds from the bowl on the bar, 'Thank you, Henry.' He nodded at the barman and left.

And now here we were, three fat men in heavy dark suits, seated at the best table in the club. Sebastian had been late, of course, short and round and anxious he might have missed the Scotch eggs.

Reggie was subdued. He was sixty-nine but, despite his height, girth and considerable bulk, his proportions gave him a vulnerable air, top heavy and teetering, like an outsized toddler. He had a very large bald head with a few grey curls brushing his ears and collar, and a rather red nose, and yet there was something rakish and debonair about his beautiful double-breasted chalk-striped suit and dainty buckled black shoes.

'I'm going on a diet,' he told us as we shook out our napkins. 'And I'd like you to join me.'

'Just before lunch?' protested Sebastian, peeved and incredulous. 'Tell me you're joking!' His pink, handsome, rather shiny face longingly tracked a plate of mini Scotch eggs being carried to a neighbouring table, and a silver sauceboat, the size of a boot, brim-full of quivering mayonnaise. 'I had my heart set on the baby Scotch eggs!'

'Not before lunch, Sebastian. Not even before Christmas,' Reggie replied testily, irked by his outrage. 'Next year.'

'What a bore!' said Sebastian. 'Why?'

Reggie's joie de vivre, generosity and appetite were legendary. The thought of him cutting down on anything seemed not only absurd but quite simply wrong. He might as well have claimed to be taking up ballet or flying to Mars. I was as fazed as Sebastian.

'Are you ill?' I asked.

'Don't think so. Unless vanity's a sickness,' he said solemnly. Otto, the club wine waiter, filled our glasses with Chablis and left the bottle on the table.

'Well?'

'They're making a series about First Eleven, a television series.' Reggie set up the charity, First Eleven, when he sold his business in 2006. It rents land from local farmers to provide temporary cricket pitches and coaching for schools without playing fields. 'It seems there's a sort of template to these programmes. They like to build the thing around a key character: me.'

'Makes sense,' Sebastian nodded. 'You did found the bloody thing, and you do run it.'

'They want me to appear in every episode. Blether on earnestly to camera. Dash about looking purposeful.'

6

'So? What's the problem?'

'I begged to be left out but they simply insist and the sponsors and other backers are adamant.'

'I'm not surprised. You were brilliant in that promotional video. Raised a fortune, didn't it?'

'Someone said I looked like a pregnant bulldog . . .'

'Everyone said you looked like a pregnant bulldog. People love pregnant bulldogs. They're good telly. That's what they want.'

'Well, it's not what I want.'

'It's your charity. If you still believe in the thing, you have to do it.'

'I'm going to do it, but not as that bloated clown in the video, that wheezing buffoon. I refuse to look that ludicrous in front of an audience of thousands.'

'Millions maybe.'

'Preserved on the web for all eternity as a panting hippopotamus.'

'I never think of you as panting particularly.'

'Thank you.'

'They say television adds ten pounds.'

'Thank you too, George. Maybe it does, but I need to lose *forty* pounds. Filming starts in five months or so. Maybe six. Five months to turn from bulldog to boxer. So I'm going on a diet and I want you to join me.'

'Very unwise to tinker with one's way of life at your age, Reggie,' Sebastian told him earnestly, clutching at straws. 'What does Jane think?'

'She's thrilled. The doctor's been nagging me to lose weight anyway. To think about losing weight for ages.'

'Have you ever been to the doctor and not been nagged about weight?' Sebastian said dismissively. 'You're happy and busy and retired, for goodness' sake. If one can't relax about the odd extra pound at seventy, when the hell can one?'

Reggie did seem to have a happy life. He had been one of the first people in Britain to get into portable loos, initially for building sites, then 'events and functions'. Gradually the business expanded into mobile offices and homes, portable everything, getting more and more luxurious each year. He sold out in 2006 and set up First Eleven, courting farmers, perfecting his mobile cricket pavilions and raising money. The charity was so effective and popular it attracted the favourable attention of the media and politicians. Rumour had it, that with First Eleven and Reggie's other charitable work, apparently no skeletons in his cupboard, and a lifetime of successful business behind him, the prime minister had plans to 'help him give something back'.

'I'm sixty-nine. Not much older than you,' Reggie retorted indignantly. Sebastian is sixty-one. I am fifty-two. 'A virtual spring chicken in this day and age,' he added, glaring defiantly at each of us in turn. 'But I *am* going to get back in shape for this bloody programme, and seeing how you two are both so . . . so . . . *mis*-shapen yourselves . . .' He glared at us again, 'Out of shape yourselves. I thought you might join me?'

He turned to a passing waiter and, in a rather less passionate tone, ordered lunch for us all.

8

'May we have a very large jug of tap water, please? And I think we'll all have the Scotch eggs and then the turkey?' He looked round for our approval. We smiled encouragingly. 'With all the trimmings.'

'May I have the potted shrimps rather than the Scotch eggs, please, Reggie?' I said.

'And I'd rather have goose instead of turkey,' said Sebastian. 'And four rather than just three Scotch eggs if possible, please?'

'Of course,' he beamed at the waiter. 'Thank you.' He turned back. 'So?' he said.

'You haven't sold it very well,' chided Sebastian, after a pause. 'Recruitment by insult is generally regarded as a bit of an oxymoron.'

The water and three toast racks were placed on the table. Sebastian hastily buttered himself a white triangle before anyone could snatch it away. 'I don't really believe in dieting anyway,' he said between munches. 'In fact, I rather disapprove.'

'Obviously!' Reggie retorted, flicking a contemptuous glance at Sebastian's midriff. 'Talking of morons.'

'You're not being entirely reasonable,' continued Sebastian, reaching for another piece of toast. 'The Grace Browns have always been big. My father and grandfather were massive: very, very big; mighty trenchermen. It's genetic.'

'So's haemophilia. Doesn't mean it's good for you.'

'But you have an incentive, Reggie. We haven't. And I'm single now, unlike you two, and – despite all the propaganda – I've come to realise that girls rather fancy a larger bloke, girls of a certain age.'

'Bollocks.'

'Shows he can bring home the bacon. It is a subconscious thing. They don't even know it themselves.'

'Ah,' Reggie nodded sarcastically. 'Hence your army of ardent admirers.'

'But that's not really the point. Chatting people up invariably involves grub, at some point. I can't nibble a celery stick while they knock back the lobster and champagne. Nothing could be more of a turn-off. *And* I feel great, health-wise, perhaps because I don't waste my time pestering doctors. Right as a trivet. What about you, George?'

'No, I don't actually,' I replied.

'Don't you?'

'I'm as fat as a pig, Sebo, let's face it, and I'd much rather not be. The waistband on this suit is like cheese wire. I have to wear a jersey now to hide the fact I can't do my trousers up properly.'

'I was wondering about the tank top. Just assumed it was an early Christmas present.'

'Fiona says I've started to snore . . . horribly. And it's really getting her down and I'm pretty sure it's a weight thing. It's . . . dispiriting. Standing on the platform at Kelvedon Station this morning I could feel the skin from my multiple chins pressing cold against each other.'

'It was freezing this morning!'

'And when I leant forward in my seat, my belly actually rested on my lap and got in the way of my forearms.'

'The seats are minuscule on those trains. *Tiny!*'

'I have moobs.'

10

'What?'

'Man boobs, a moon face and my mind hasn't caught up and still thinks I'm gorgeous.'

'What's wrong with that?'

'I get a jolt every time I see my reflection. Frankly, I'm downright obese and I've got to do something about it. So I'm in. Count me in, Reggie. And of course you'll do it too, Sebo.'

'Well of course,' he grumbled, 'having no mind of my own.' He poured himself another glass of wine and took a hearty gulp. 'But not because I'm kowtowing to the health zealots, but because I'm wet, too wet to say no to my friends.' He was momentarily distracted by the arrival of the Scotch eggs, but continued ranting on in autopilot as we waited for the mayonnaise and my shrimps. 'It's all a government conspiracy, anyway, this obsession with weight . . .'

'Yes, yes, of course,' Reggie shushed.

'. . . to make everyone so morose and miserable, so used to life by diktat, that we don't object, don't even notice, their creeping encroachments on our ancient liberties. Too fixated with our earthly bodies to fight for our eternal souls!' A waitress brought my potted shrimps and another placed a huge silver sauceboat on the table. Sebastian's eyes locked onto it. 'May I have some mayonnaise, please?' he said.

'So that's a yes, then, Sebo? Well. Thank you,' Reggie said, grinning suddenly and passing the silver jug. He chortled to himself for a second, then picked up his knife and fork and, having subjected a Scotch egg to a series of minute adjustments, plunged his blade through the crust. Something very like molten butter erupted from the breach, then oozed over the bread-crumbed surface: perhaps simply pure fat.

'The New Year, you say?' Sebastian continued. 'You're giving us Christmas to get used to the idea?'

'Mentally prepare yourselves, yes, and do your research.' Reggie took a succulent mouthful of meat smothered in mayonnaise and executed an exquisite slow-motion crunch. He held the piping hot morsel on his tongue with his mouth slightly open, and exhaled slowly to cool the gobbet, emitting a momentary wisp of steam before swallowing. Then he nodded, mumbling dreamily. 'Gosh that was . . . good.'

'No wonder they call it the mother sauce,' said Sebastian, already on his second dollop. 'This mayonnaise is sensational. And very easy to make, apparently.'

'Aren't there five mother sauces?' I mused. 'I seem to remember one of them is tomato.'

'According to who?' Reggie asked.

'The Hairy Bikers of course,' said Sebastian. 'Do you think there is some sort of link between cooking and motorbikes? The Two Fat Ladies had a bike too.'

'Just one?'

'That can't be true?'

'Yes. A Triumph Thunderbird and sidecar.' Sebastian had a Kawasaki.

'No, I mean the mother sauces and the Hairy Bikers. I had no idea they were so influential.'

'They're not. It was the Frogs, you plonker. The French. I forget how gullible you are. Rather adorable really.'

12

'Thanks.'

'And George is right. One of the five French mother sauces is made from tomato, and three from flour and various stocks: veal, fish, beef. But the mother of the mothers, in my eyes, the *grand-mère*, has got to be mayonnaise. And its derivatives and variations; emulsions of egg yolk and butter or oil: hollandaise, Béarnaise, et cetera. Different names, different flavours and textures, but essentially the same sauce.'

'Hollandaise? As in Holland? Hang on, I thought it was French,' said Reggie.

'Created by French Huguenots returning to France from exile in Protestant Holland. Mayonnaise isn't Spanish either.'

'Why should it be?'

'It's named after Mahón in Menorca.'

'Is Menorca in Spain?'

'Yes. Some French admiral captured it and the only things left to eat were eggs and olive oil. His chef whipped them up together and *voilà*! Mahón or mayon-naise.'

'I love mayonnaise,' I said, 'but I'm not sure I could eat it on its own.'

'Groaning with bloody calories of course,' said Sebastian, before cramming in a forkful of Scotch egg, having dunked it in his dollop, and chewing with brisk deliberation.

'You mentioned research, Reggie,' he said after swallowing. 'What do you mean, research?' But Reggie was still savouring our recruitment.

'I *am* glad you're both on board,' he said, looking up from his plate and beaming at us each in turn. 'I thought I might have to ask Geoffrey.'

13

'Geoffrey?'

'Geoffrey Bramley.' Geoffrey was the Master of our local beagle pack, the Essex Foot.

'Why?'

'Put on a huge amount of weight when he was laid up with that ingrowing toenail. Can't keep up with the hounds any more, and of course refuses to use a quad bike or pony.'

'Well, it is the Essex *Foot*, after all. But he's not the easiest chap in the world.'

'That's what Jane said. She suggested I join Weight Watchers, if you said no.'

'Weight Watchers?' Sebastian blurted, fork halfway to his mouth again. He actually put the fork down, still laden. 'Do you like being watched?'

'It is not about being watched, Sebastian,' Reggie assured him. 'Or at least not in a negative sense. More about joint watching; self-watching.'

'That's what the Stasi said.'

'It's about mutual support, team effort, watching each other's backs. You're all in it together, but of course much more fun with old friends.'

'Hate teams, always have,' said Sebastian. 'Stag parties, hooligans, lynch mobs. Perhaps because I'm crap at games? Too competitive.'

'That doesn't make sense.'

'I'm so competitive I can't bear not to win. So I refuse to play at all: "I strove with none for none were worth my strife."'

'Who said that?'

'Forgotten. Byron, I think.'

'Keen cricketer, Byron.'

'Was he?'

'Always dieting.'

'Bit of a tit, Byron. Maybe it was Landor. But tell me about this research, Reggie?'

'You've just made my point with your teams. We need a plan, Sebastian. We *each* need our *own* plan. Weight Watchers provides a plan – a very simple, proven plan – based on calories, I think, but teams aren't your cup of tea so it's not for you. You'll come up with a different plan having done your research. We're each different.'

'Of course,' conceded Sebastian. 'You're going to use the word "lifestyle" next, I can sense it.' Reggie ignored him.

'Can you remember George's sponsored diet, when he lost all that weight for the cottage hospital?' He turned to me. 'What was it, George? Two stone in twelve weeks?'

'Thirty pounds,' I admitted.

'But three months later you were back where you started, weren't you?'

'Not quite . . . but pretty much.'

'And now you're even bigger? Fat as a pig, you said?' I poured myself some tap water and took a sip of wine.

'Yes,' I conceded.

'Well, that's crazy! That's why we need a long-term plan, a "lifestyle" plan, to get the weight off and keep it off . . .' Reggie symbolically pushed the mayonnaise jug away and thoughtfully helped himself to a final triangle of toast. '. . . after all that self-denial. Otherwise the whole thing's pointless.'

15

'I thought this was about looking good on telly? Not a career with the Chippendales.'

'There's no point losing it just to put it back on again.'

'How much are you aiming to lose?' I asked warily.

'Enough to look half human again. My GP said one should aim for the recommended BMI. That people who weigh what they should, look as they should.'

'Glib bastard. Some people are just plain ugly,' Sebastian observed, 'whatever they weigh, and most of them perfectly happy, decent people too. And, anyway, recommended by whom?'

'Oh, I don't know. Doctors I suppose.'

'And what is the BMI? More medical mumbo-jumbo.'

'Come on, Sebastian. Do try to be a bit more positive. Your girls thought you might want to get trim for the wedding. Don't you want to look your best in the photographs?' Sebastian's eldest daughter Natasha was getting married in May.

'Depends how you define best. Take Fat Jack in the hall: *that* was gorgeous in 1810. Until Beau Brummell came along and ruined it all.'

'How did Beau Brummell ruin it all?'

'One of the first full-time trendsetters: he was a narcissist obsessed with cravat knots.'

'What?'

'You know, cravat knots. Like tie knots.'

'Oh.'

'Utter show-off. Striking "attitudes" in the bow window at White's so everyone could admire his sublime new togs and "sporting figure" as they plodded up and down St James's. Had himself publicly weighed once a week on the scales at Berry Brothers: vanity personified. It was he who invented dreary trousers, with a strap under the boot, instead of good old britches. Had calves like Twiglets, apparently. The original fat-ist.'

'Well, I suppose we all have our issues,' Reggie said generously.

'He got his comeuppance in the end.'

'How?'

'He was best buddies with the Prince Regent, the future George IV, the frustrated chubster who built Brighton. His sort of favourite.'

'And?'

'They had a row about something or other?'

'Cravat knots?'

'Do you know, Reggie, I think it was. Anyway the Prince Regent bumped into him somewhere or other and cut him dead. Brummell turned to the prince's equerry and asked loudly, "And who's your fat friend?" That was that. Ostracised by the whole of London and died in penury and disgrace.'

'The perfect reason for preferring Fat Jack's kind of gorgeous,' I said. 'Though I bet he snored like a pig.'

'Who?'

'Fat Jack.'

'Snoring was the least of his wife's problems, by the look of him. He must have weighed thirty stone. But I do get George's point,' Sebastian conceded. 'There's something particularly tragic about pissing someone off while you're fast asleep. It got Mary down.'

Sebastian and his wife Mary separated five years ago. She still lives in their old home a few miles from us in Essex. Sebastian moved back to London, into a friend's ground-floor flat near Sloane Square. The friend, the landlord, on holiday in Goa for the last forty years, insists on no repairs or refurbishment and the right to move back in at one week's notice. Accordingly the rent is absurdly 'reasonable' but the flat is rather a dump.

Sebastian has a small gallery specialising in animal oils near Christie's, packed with beautiful things, most of which he is notoriously reluctant to sell; as his wife is said to have 'got everything' in their divorce, he is widely assumed to be broke.

'Fiona tells me it gets especially bad when I reach about fourteen stone, around the fifth hole in my belt.'

'So you need to get back to the fourth hole in your belt? Are you wearing it now?'

'No, braces.'

'If you were, which hole would you be on?'

'The eighth.'

'So you need to lose four holes.'

'He needs to lose *six* holes,' Reggie insisted. 'And stay there.' He smiled at the waiters clearing our plates. 'Fiona told Jane that being in bed with you, George, is like sleeping in a drum . . .' Our wives, Fiona, Jane and Mary, have been neighbours and friends for twenty-five years. ' . . . a giant drum being rolled down a cobbled street.'

'She told me that too.'

'But it's not just the snoring: it's health generally. The fact is that being overweight is bad for you, very bad indeed. And as we get older, we have less and less time to rectify the situation. So we've got to overshoot, then the occasional relapse won't matter.'

'Great,' Sebastian muttered, half under his breath. 'You've become a fanatic.'

'Yes, *great*, Sebastian. And once we get there we can ease off, once we've stabilised. But not too quickly either, or the skin can't cope. Look at poor Colonel Derek over there.' He jerked his head at the club table, where a gaunt old man, short and enwizened, was eating on his own, a copy of *Marie Claire* propped open on a bookstand in front of him. 'Lost so much weight after his wife left that the skin was hanging down in swags like Ali Baba's trousers. Eventually they cut a three-foot strip off his waist and he had it made into a gun-sleeve.'

'What a good idea,' said Sebastian. 'Though there does still seem to be a bit of . . . slack?'

'You mean the wattles? The empty jowls?'

'Certainly a wallet. Maybe even a cartridge bag? Is it true he's got a gastric band?'

'So everyone says, but I don't think we're quite there yet, are we? The gastric-band stage? Let's try dieting first. We need to sort out a strategy. Not too fast, not too slow, just right.'

'The Goldilocks Diet.'

'I heard somewhere or other that one should aim to lose one, one and a half pounds a week.'

'You'll be on it for ever then, Reggie.'

'Filming's due to start in late May, early June.'

'That *is* for ever.'

'Five months or so. Let's say twenty weeks at one and a half pounds a week.' I calculated. 'Thirty pounds. That's over two stone.'

'Five months?' Sebastian said flatly. 'Nearly half a year.'

'And whether to cut calories or carbs? All these things have to be considered.'

'What precisely *is* a carb?' asked Sebastian, trying to be positive. 'Or a calorie, for that matter?'

'Do you really not know?' Reggie exclaimed. 'I thought you went to Oxford?'

'Why should I know?' demanded Sebastian, fat from the Scotch eggs glistening on his chin. 'I read history, not nutrition.' He wiped his chin with a napkin.

'It's bread and potatoes and pasta and rice . . .'

'You're telling me a loaf is a carb? A potato is a carb?'

'No, no, of course not. But they contain carbs.'

'So what is a carb then? I thought you went to Gordonstoun? Look it up on your telephone.'

'I can't. I'm on the committee,' Reggie hissed, looking round furtively. 'But as the name suggests, a carbohydrate is a combination of carbon and hydrogen . . .' As he faltered, Otto placed a *Pocket Oxford English Dictionary* on the table beside him. 'Thank you, Otto,' Reggie said smoothly. 'This'll get it exactly.' He flicked the pages. 'Ah. Here we are: *Carbohydrate: energy-producing organic compound of carbon with oxygen and hydrogen: starch, sugar, glucose.*'

'I see,' said Sebastian. 'And bread, potatoes and pasta are all full of them?' Reggie nodded encouragingly. 'And sugar?' Sebastian thought for a moment. 'So carbs are basically what make food worth eating?' Silence. 'What's a calorie then?'

Reggie turned back a few pages and read on.

'*Unit of quantity of heat. Amount of heat required to raise the temperature of one gram of water one degree centigrade. Accordingly used to express the energy value of foods.*'

'Very much like a carb then,' said Sebastian. 'This is going to be fun.'

'Not fun, Sebo, but *good*. Because making things better *is* good. And it's simple. We just cut out pudding, potatoes and pasta and the weight pours off. And port, I suppose.'

'The Begins with a Bloody P Diet.'

'I don't see why you are making such a fuss about it, Sebo,' said Reggie, genuinely bemused. 'You just eat less and perhaps move a bit more: basic physics. Burn more calories than you take on board. And gradually turn into a very much healthier, better-looking man.'

'And I can't understand why you don't see what a big deal this is. You're asking me to completely change my life for months. Half a year. Half a year without all the things that make food enjoyable, edible even! And I like the way I look. And it's all right for you two. You live in the sticks miles from anywhere. You have literally zero temptation. Other than the odd pub and takeaway, there are what? Maybe three decent restaurants in the whole of East Anglia?'

'Don't be ridiculous.'

'I live here! London! Currently the culinary centre of the universe. With nothing to keep me in my, let's be honest, cramped and shabby flat, but a farting lodger and my *Game of Thrones* box set. On the other side of my door, every day, every night, there's glorious, busy London, teeming with stunning single women and at least 40,000 restaurants to take them to. It's . . . it's irresistible. I'm going to have to chain myself to the radiator like Jason and his flipping Argonauts.'

'Only for a few months.'

'Exactly.' Sebastian looked appalled. In his distress he scanned the table for anything else to eat, realised there was nothing and started wringing his napkin, more pink and cherubic than ever.

'I do appreciate your help with all this, Sebo,' Reggie said gently. 'I'm sorry it seems such an ordeal.'

Otto placed a decanted magnum of Rioja on the table, with the cork tucked into the rim of the coaster, paused for a moment to allow us to admire it, then poured a splash into Reggie's glass. He took a deep sniff and nodded. 'Perfect, Otto. Thank you.' Otto filled our glasses.

'Only wankers know anything about wine,' Sebastian growled when Otto had gone.

'Otto's one of my best friends!' Reggie spluttered, flushing crimson.

'I didn't mean Otto.'

'Ah.' Reggie scowled, colour fading. 'Well, here's the goose and turkey.' And indeed here they were, with roast potatoes like gleaming nuggets of crackling, parsnips, lightly steamed Brussels sprouts drenched in butter, bread sauce, cranberry sauce, two sorts of stuffing and gravy. We tucked in with gusto, grunting with satisfaction and passing the sauces to and fro.

Reggie was the first to push his plate away, using both hands to refill our glasses from the magnum rather than wait for Otto.

'I like a magnum,' said Sebastian. 'Shows commitment. Perfectly happy to have a bottle of wine at lunch,' he grinned. 'But I'd much rather have two. It never occurred to me Rioja came in magnums. What a happy thing.'

'What's the next one up?' I asked. 'Four bottles?'

'Yes, the double magnum or Jeroboam: "the mighty man of valour who made Israel to sin".'

'Then ten bottles?'

'Decimal? Are you joking?' I lowered my eyes. 'Six bottles: Rehoboam, after the son of Solomon, King of Israel, who said, "My father chastised you with whips but I shall chastise you with scorpions!" That's what I call a manifesto.'

'What's a Balthazar then?'

'Sixteen bottles, after Nebuchadnezzar's son, who was weighed in the balance and found wanting.'

'Sounds more like our man,' said Reggie.

'He was slain by Darius the Mede.' Sebastian put his glass to his lips with surprising delicacy and then held the wine in his mouth for a moment before swallowing. 'It really is good, Reggie. Fit for the Infanta of Spain. Made from the "noble grape", tempranillo, brought to Spain by the Phoenicians.'

'So the Phoenicians reached Spain?'

'They not only reached it, they named it. "Spain" comes from the Phoenician for "the land of the rabbit". We should really be having this with *lapin à la cocotte*.'

'I thought only wankers knew anything about wine,' Reggie observed.

'Sorry,' said Sebastian. 'This whole diet thing has knocked me for six a bit.'

'I should have warned you.' Reggie took a solemn sip of wine himself, apology accepted. 'Are we all happy to meet here again at the end of the first fortnight in January?' He carefully set the glass back down. 'For another lunch and second weigh-in on the boot-room scales?'

'When's the first weigh-in?' asked Sebastian, not quite finished.

'Now.'

'What?'

'Today. After lunch.'

'*What*? But that's bonkers, Reggie! Everyone always doubles in size over Christmas, especially me. I'm spending it with the girls and the food will be out of this world.' By the girls he meant his ex-wife and two grown-up daughters. 'I assumed ... The New Year ... Reggie ... Please?'

'I'm sorry, Sebo, but that's precisely why I want to start now. I need to get a grip straight away – this evening, in fact. You kick off when you like but we all get weighed today. If we have the next meeting in mid-Jan, you'll have plenty of time to get a bit of traction after the New Year.'

'Well, in that case I'm bloody well making hay while the sun shines. I'll have brandy-butter ice cream with my Christmas pud and mince pies, *and* brandy butter. And then perhaps a squint at the cheeseboard.' He looked round determinedly. 'And a glass of that very good madeira.'

'You don't even like Christmas pud.'

'Says who?'

'Says me. You only have it once a year.'

'Rubbish. I had it three times last week.'

'Christmas pudding was just a practical solution to a medieval problem; when they had to slaughter spare livestock before winter to conserve fodder, they preserved the meat with dried fruit in a pastry shell.'

'So?'

'It's completely obsolete, like Spam or bread and dripping. If you like it so much, why do you only have it at Christmas time?'

'Because there are a thousand other puddings to have at other times, but Christmas time is the time for Christmas pud.'

'Hmmph. Well, they've run out of the madeira.'

When lunch was over, Reggie led the way right down to the boot room.

'I'll join you there.' Sebastian waved us on. 'I've just got to have a quick word with the porters.'

In between old photographs and racing prints, the boot room seemed to be walled with mahogany, the doors of lockers and loos, and bristling with rank upon rank of brass hooks. It was dank and battered and due for its first overhaul in decades that Christmas. Against one wall stood the vast Victorian scales, perhaps originally designed for weighing jockeys, consisting principally of an upholstered bench on a wooden plinth, with a brass, clock-like dial to one side. Henry the barman placed a calculator and a leather folder on the counter under the skylight. Reggie opened the folder and removed a piece of dye-stamped club writing paper. Folding it in half lengthways and then in half again, he created four columns. He took a pen like a gold zeppelin from his jacket and wrote our names across the top in the second, third and fourth columns, in order of age, then the date on the line below, in the first column.

Sebastian joined us, with the final glass of Rioja, looking strangely hunched and dishevelled.

'What's the calculator for?' he asked suspiciously.

'To calculate our BMIs,' Reggie said.

Henry approached the scales, grabbed a large brass knob and forced it sharply down, freeing the bench, which now visibly trembled and wobbled.

Reggie took off his jacket and hung it on a peg, then sat carefully on the scales. Henry peered at the dial.

'Two and a quarter hundredweight, or 252 pounds,' Henry intoned. 'Dead on eighteen stone, sir.'

'Bloody Nora!' gasped Sebastian. 'What a whopper.'

'Are you sure, Henry?' Reggie squeaked, leaping off as though stung and quite clearly aghast. 'That's way more than I was this morning!'

'It must be the shoes, sir,' Henry assured him. 'Try again without the shoes.'

I looked at the dial. 'It's not set to nought,' I said. 'We need to twizzle this cog, I think.' We twizzled, bringing the single arm back from eight pounds to zero.

Reggie bent and unlaced his shoes, took them off, sat down, plonk, on the bench again, eyes straight ahead, hands on knees, holding his breath.

'Seventeen stone and six pounds,' read Henry.

'Fractionally better, I suppose,' Reggie said with a sigh. 'Can you convert that into kilos for me, please, Henry?'

'Why? What's wrong with stones and pounds?' demanded Sebastian sharply.

'I can only do the BMI calculation in metric.'

Henry tapped at the calculator.

'That's 110.7 kilos, sir.'

Sebastian trudged to the scales and sat down.

'Seventeen stone one pound,' read Henry. 'Which is 108.4 kilos.'

'Impossible,' Reggie said kindly. 'Try without your jacket.' He reached for Sebastian's lapel but Sebastian flinched away, his bulging pockets actually thunking against the scales. Reggie looked puzzled and then suspicious.

'What have you got in your jacket, Sebastian? What *have* you got in your pockets?'

'Nothing,' Sebastian said weakly, 'much.'

Reggie reached into one of Sebastian's pockets and with some difficulty drew out what looked like a large lead turd, obviously very heavy. He placed it on the counter behind him, shaking his head with disappointment. After a moment Sebastian took something similar from his other pocket. Each had an iron ring at one end.

'What on earth are they?' Reggie sighed.

27

'The weights from the hall clock,' admitted Sebastian. 'Sorry.' He got off the scales and hung up his jacket. 'But I told you this is my busy time of year: shoots and dinner parties and whatnot. Christmas lunch, for goodness' sake, and New Year's Eve! You haven't really given us time.' Reggie set his jaw, not to be mollified. 'So I thought I'd help it along with a bit of extra ballast at the start, so I could make an initial dent in the thing on the second weighing, without necessarily being too scrupulous over the hols.'

'George, your turn,' Reggie said, tight-lipped.

I took off my jacket but kept on my shoes and lowered myself gingerly on to the leather.

'Fifteen stone seven pounds,' Henry said, matter-of-factly. I couldn't help glancing at the dial. 'I checked it was back at nought, sir,' he said, reading my mind. 'That is 98.4 kilos.'

'Blimey!' I said, surprised and appalled.

'Very heavy cloth that.' Reggie tried to cushion the blow. 'And you've still got your shoes on.'

'And your watch,' Sebastian said meekly.

'Shall we try you again, Sebo? *If* you've had enough time?' Reggie said sarcastically.

Colonel Derek strutted down the stairs and marched on the urinals.

Sebastian approached the scales once more. Sitting on the bench with his hands in his lap, feet swinging.

'Don't swing your feet,' Reggie ordered.

'Fifteen stone nine pounds.'

'Rubbish!' snapped Sebastian, dismounting and puffing as he unlaced his shoes.

'Ninety-nine point three kilos,' said Henry.

Once Sebastian's shoes were off, he got on again: still fifteen stone nine.

'Impossible, Henry, I'm thirteen stone. Always have been. The shoes must weigh something!' Sebastian softly placed his shoes on the scales and stepped back, scrutinising the dial. It had not moved. 'Do you think a dump would make any difference?'

'I used to enjoy a good shit,' said the colonel, washing his hands with a bar of amber soap.

'Bloody hell!' fumed Sebastian. 'I'm vast.'

Henry carefully wrote down Sebastian's weight in stones and pounds, and kilos, on the sheet.

'In training?' asked the colonel.

'Dieting,' I told him.

'Shed a few pounds myself.' He sidled towards us and lowered his voice. 'Did you know that for every two and a half stone you lose, your cock gets a quarter-inch longer?'

'Hardly seems worth it,' Sebastian spluttered.

'Point six three five centimetres,' Henry intoned, with a straight face.

'Bloody Europe,' said Sebastian.

'Well, I won't be betting on you, Brown,' wattled the tiny colonel, suddenly furious, 'having seen you at lunch.'

'Won't you?' Sebastian snapped back, bright pink from lacing his shoes and the realisation of quite how heavy he was. 'I'll give you a pound a pound.'

'Over how long?'

'Five months.'

'Six. Possibly,' Reggie said hurriedly. 'Not entirely certain yet.'

'One hundred pounds,' the colonel retorted.

'What do you mean?'

'One hundred pounds a pound.'

'Don't be ridiculous,' Sebastian told him.

'Ten then,' said the colonel. 'Ten pounds to you for every pound you lose. Ten pounds to me for every pound you gain. Lambert to invigilate and call time.'

'Done,' said Sebastian, holding out his hand.

'I don't shake hands,' said the colonel, turning away for a final glance in the mirror. He straightened his tie, favoured us all with a faint nod and left.

'There's something very unlikable about that man,' Sebastian said.

'Now for the science,' said Reggie. 'What are your heights?'

Reggie worked out our BMIs by dividing our weight in kilograms by the square of our heights in metres.

'So at 110.7 kilos and six foot three inches, that's 75 inches times 2.54, which makes 190.5 centimetres, or 1.905 metres, times 1.905, which equals 3.629025. So that's 110.7 divided by 3.629025.'

'Fuck, this is complicated!' Sebastian blurted, still fuming at the colonel.

'That's a BMI of 30.5: just obese.'

'I should think you bloody well are after all that!'

Reggie ignored him. 'But I should be a maximum of fourteen stone, to have a BMI of 25. So I need to lose three stone six pounds. At least forty-eight pounds at one and a half pounds a week, that's thirty-two weeks or eight months. I'll do it in the five.'

30

'Is that what we're aiming for? A BMI of 25?'

'Well, according to the doc, one's BMI should be between 18.5 and 25.'

'Well, what about me then?' asked Sebastian, curious despite himself.

Reggie tapped the calculator and made notes on the back of his hand. 'You're obese too: your BMI is 32. Your target's eleven and a half stone. Four stone to lose: nine months. George? You're not quite so bad. BMI of 29.6: simply overweight. At the very top end of overweight: only three stone to lose. On the bright side, according to my chart, none of us is morbidly obese.'

'*Morbidly* obese? Who coins these phrases?' Sebastian asked, suddenly dejected, almost physically deflated.

'Shall I write the targets down too?' asked Reggie. 'So we know what we're aiming for?'

'If you must,' Sebastian sighed.

Henry passed the folder to Reggie who wrote in the targets, signed the page with a flourish and stowed it in his pocket.

Henry snapped the empty folder shut and returned to the bar. We put our jackets and shoes back on. Reggie passed the clock weights to Sebastian. We filed after Henry and watched Sebastian re-hang the weights, correct the time, and set the pendulum swinging again. Then Sebastian ordered three double espressos and a jug of hot milk.

'We should have a photograph,' said Reggie, brandishing his mobile. 'Before and after, while Henry's making the coffee. Let's ask Mustafa.'

The duty porter was only too happy to oblige. We trooped outside then he, resplendent in his dark green tailcoat, brilliant brass buttons and faded gold braid, tried to chivvy us all into shot.

'Say cheese,' he said.

'Don't they say sausages nowadays?' Reggie asked.

'I thought they said prune,' said Sebastian.

'Who?'

'People who get photographed a lot. Celebrities. According to my daughters.'

'Celebrities?' demanded an urgent female voice, possibly Australian, and we noticed a couple, dressed for hill walking, peering at us over Mustafa's shoulder. 'Who are they?' The man took off his glasses and peered harder.

'No one,' he replied, putting his glasses back on and turning away. 'Just three fat drongos.'

CHAPTER 2

'He hath filled the hungry with good things; and the
rich he hath sent empty away.'

Luke 1:51, *The King James Bible*

We had agreed on fortnightly weigh-ins, but it was not until the
third week of January that we met at the Spatchcock again, at
eight in the morning.

Reggie and I had both been rather irritated by Sebastian's
insistence on treating us all to a pub breakfast. Not only did we
have to get up at five thirty in Essex to be in St James's by eight,
but neither of us wanted to have our self-control blown out of
the water by exposure to Sebastian enjoying a 'full English'.

It was so early the porter had to unlock the front door. The
boot room had been redecorated between Christmas and the
New Year and, as soon as we reached the head of the stairs, we
could smell the fresh paint like the first day of term. The walls
were now a sort of surgical mushroom colour, the stone floor
repointed, the wood varnished and the brass gleaming. Many of
the racing prints and photographs had been reframed and all

had been rearranged, leaving a large space high up in the middle of the wall. The chrome work on the sinks beneath – and on the elephantine urinals – shone like platinum; the bars of soap had been replaced with amber squirter bottles, and even the towels were new. It was almost too pristine and clinical, like a modern hotel, except for the worn red leather and tarnished dial of the colossal Victorian scales.

Reggie ceremoniously smoothed our page open on the counter and one by one we took our seats on the bench: he had lost over a stone, sixteen pounds, in what was effectively three weeks. I had lost just under a stone, twelve pounds, in two, and Sebastian had lost five pounds.

Reggie duly noted the results on a fresh line.

'What's that in metric?' Sebastian whooped.

'Quite a lot,' said Reggie with quiet satisfaction. 'Really rather a lot.' But if Reggie was smug, Sebastian was euphoric.

'Five pounds.' He laughed. 'Incredible. That's almost half a stone. Piece of cake!' He drew himself up as straight as he could, sucking his stomach in and looking at himself sideways in the full-length mirror. 'So much for one pound a week. Though I am aching with hunger. You've done brilliantly, Reggie.'

'Apparently it's normal to lose a lot at the start,' Reggie said modestly, embarrassed by his success. 'Water retention or something.'

'Can't apply to me,' said Sebastian. 'Never touch the stuff . . . neat.'

The colonel stomped down the stairs, flung his overcoat and trilby on a peg and marched on the urinals.

'What are you doing here so damned early?' he growled.

'Weighing ourselves,' said Sebastian smugly. 'I've lost five pounds.'

'We'll see,' grunted the colonel. 'Quaking in my boots.'

'What are *you* doing here so damned early?'

'Collecting my port. Been saving it for the right moment. Thought it might go down well with the Senile Delinquents.' The Spatchcock held free quarterly lunches for members over seventy-five, or who had been in the club for fifty years or more. It was said, in the light of their age, that you never sat next to the same person twice. 'But the wine committee has become the investment committee, and they don't want it.'

'What?'

'Not a good investment, calculating bastards. Even for nothing. Though they're happy to sell it, of course, and trouser the takings. Health and safety won't allow "anything not purchased and maintained by qualified cellarage personnel".'

'Surely Otto's not in on this?'

'Of course not. Outsourced to some frightful consultants.'

'By who?'

'The chairman. Pinion.'

'And he's making you take it away again?'

'He was going to charge me for leaving it here! I was trying to give them a present, not hire storage space. Fuck him!'

'That's unbelievable,' said Reggie. 'I'm . . . sorry.'

The colonel did not reply. He seemed to be having difficulty peeing.

'What do you think of the revamp?' Sebastian asked.

35

'Terrible!' The colonel snarled over his shoulder, gasping with concentration. 'Makes your cock look so shabby.' After a few agonising seconds he jerked his flies shut and advanced on the sinks as though to rip them from the wall. 'And what are they putting up there?' He gestured at the gap in the racing prints above the mirror. 'Strictures on personal hygiene, no doubt, or a bloody great "no wanking" sign.' He dried his hands on a linen napkin and dashed it into an open laundry basket before fuming back upstairs muttering. We followed meekly in his wake and shambled out.

'I'm worried about Pinion. Very worried,' said Reggie.

'Join the club,' said Sebastian.

'Snubbing poor old Derek like that.'

'Downright spiteful.'

'No, Sebo. Not spite, health and safety. Nothing personal about it. That's his problem, totally impersonal. Hasn't he told you about his razor-sharp business brain? It's all about numbers for him, not people. He's trying to maximise . . . whatnot.'

'You're quoting his letter. Ghastly. But personally I'm more worried by the bit on cancelling life memberships. Virtually accused us of ripping off the club.'

'I did see that. I forgot you were a life member.'

'My uncle bought it for me when Natasha got her scholarship. I couldn't afford the subs now otherwise. He'd very kindly offered to pay some of the school fees, and when that wasn't necessary any longer, sweetly made me a life member here. I used the money Mary and I'd stashed to buy the Ford Capri Ghia.'

'Mary loved that car.'

36

'So did I.'

'Don't worry, Pinion'll never get it past the committee. The club needed your money then and life means life.'

'Good. Where would I get my free Twiglets?'

Having no bedrooms, the Spatchcock did not do breakfast. Sebastian had booked a table at the Cock and Bull, and after a short walk he ushered us inside, joshing and joking with the staff and other customers.

'I hadn't expected you to be on quite such fighting form,' Reggie conceded. 'Being on a diet obviously agrees with you.'

'It's the prospect of bloody grub that agrees with me! Would warm the cockles of anyone's heart after what I endured yesterday. I'm starving.'

'Diddums.'

'But I'm coping, as I said earlier. I did my research, just as you instructed, found the least intolerable of a pretty grim and surprisingly contradictory bunch, and I'm sticking to it ... But there's something else making me cheerful: a picture, a perfect picture.' He leant forward and lowered his voice. 'Wedding present for Natasha and Milo.'

'What of?' asked Reggie.

'Great big pastel of their college from the Backs, with a couple on the bridge. Victorian. Unframed. Lovely.' Natasha, Sebastian's eldest daughter, had met her boyfriend, Milo, at Cambridge. They were due to be married there in May.

'Who's it by?'

'No signature or title, thank goodness, or the college would have clocked it. Needs a bit of a clean. Catalogued as *Period*

Couple on Bridge. Superb. It's coming up this afternoon. Auction in Salisbury: hardly anyone at the viewing. It's mine. That's why I insisted on breakfast.'

'I thought you were just being a cheapskate.'

'That too of course.' Sebastian turned to me, buzzing with excitement, wanting everyone to be happy. 'And the fact that I knew I'd be *starving*!' The pastry trolley clanked and tinkled past and his gaze caressed the contents for a moment before he tore his attention back to me. 'How's the head-hunting, George? "Big dicks" still swinging?'

'Always,' I sighed. 'But just at the moment . . .'

'What?'

'I'm more concerned with a possible balls-up.'

'What kind of balls-up?'

'Ludo.'

'The game?'

'The graduate.'

'What do you mean?'

'An old friend, marooned in the wilds of Scotland, asked me to persuade my best client to give his son a few weeks' London work experience.'

'An internship,' said Reggie.

'Doesn't internship mean unpaid?' Sebastian said.

'In this case, yes. But I was rather hoping that it might turn into the real thing . . . if he did well.'

'But Ludo hasn't covered himself in glory?' Reggie guessed.

'Well if the poor wally isn't paid . . .' Sebastian pointed out.

'I'm more worried about what I'll end up covered in.'

38

'Is it ...?' Reggie jerked his head sideways in the vague direction of the Fletcher Building on the other side of Green Park. I nodded.

'So that was *him*. I heard about the diesel,' said Reggie. 'And the other disasters.' Ludo had put diesel in the managing director's petrol car. I paled.

'He's a hyper-intelligent, really sweet boy. Got a first from Imperial. But when it comes to the workplace, he seems to have some sort of social disorder. Getting in the way, putting his foot in it. Generally pissing everyone off.'

'You won't have to worry about him for long,' said Sebastian, with annoying complacency. 'I know the type. He'll be sacked or quit in a day or two. Some people are just too bright for the real world.'

'Now I feel much better, Sebo. Thank you.'

'Talking of feeling better,' he said. 'Feast your eyes on these menus. For goodness' sake let's get our orders in.'

It was still only eight thirty and the place was packed, predominantly with men. The room was large but low and dark, with broad oak floorboards and small windows. Delicious noises and smells wafted over us from the kitchen doors to the side of the brick fireplace. Sebastian snapped his menu shut after no more than a glance, while Reggie and I scoured ours for the least fattening alternatives.

'The breakfast here was voted best in London by the Taxi Drivers' Association last year. I've been coming for ever. I sold the landlord a picture – where is it? he's moved it – that picture: the lovely naïve bull with a giant cockerel on its back, about twenty years ago.'

'But that's the pub sign.'

'He had it copied for the pub sign, yes.'

'That was a find.'

'Not exactly. I saw him mooning over it in the street several times when I'd almost despaired of selling the thing. It was just the bull then, but rather splendid. I thought it might appeal to some nice philistine from the City. You know: all that bull and bear crap they used to bang on about? After two or three extended loiters he came in and asked the price. Too much, he said. Simply couldn't afford it. Then he came back yet again and again said no. If only there was a cock in it, he said, he could justify it to his accountant. I can have a cock added, I told him, and did so quick as a flash. Took it round and hung it before he could reconsider: he paid me in eggs, bacon and coffee over three years.'

'What are the boiled eggs like?' Reggie asked doubtfully, still scanning the menu.

'Like every other boiled egg, I presume,' Sebastian replied. 'But I'll be gutted if you have a boiled egg, Reggie. This place does the best breakfast in London and therefore probably the world: centuries of wisdom and expertise distilled into one sublime culinary experience. Don't blow it on a boiled egg. It's like going to Savile Row and buying a sock.'

The publican bustled over, looking like a pantomime farmer with Dickensian side-whiskers, pink shirt, yellow waistcoat, forget-me-not corduroy trousers and beautifully polished brogues, almost as brown and shiny as his face.

'Good morning, Sebastian.' He chortled. 'No need to ask what you're having. The same for your friends?'

40

'Almost certainly not, Robert, sadly. They're dieting.'

'That is sad news.' The proprietor frowned.

'So are you, Sebo,' Reggie protested, 'in case you've forgotten. How on earth can you be having what you normally have?'

'Having done my research,' Sebastian insisted calmly, 'I've identified a system that allows me a pretty free rein as long as I stick to certain rules.'

'That makes sense,' clucked the landlord approvingly. 'Everything in moderation.' He produced a notebook and pencil from a waistcoat pocket. 'So what about you gents?' He licked the end of his pencil. 'We have exceptional kippers as usual, nothing less fattening than a nice bit of fish, and then of course there's our kedgeree. The best in London, though I say so myself, and under five hundred calories a portion. And I'm talking generous portions.'

'You're very well informed, Robert.' Sebastian sounded disappointed.

'Part of the job, Sebastian. You wouldn't believe who's counting the calories these days. Even old Arnie's turned vegetarian.'

'Has he really?' Sebastian was shocked.

'I'll have the kedgeree then, please,' said Reggie, rather warily. 'But no butter or cream.'

'Not possible, sir. Can't make kedgeree without butter or cream, I'm afraid, or not what *we* call kedgeree. Clive of India's favourite. Used to cheer himself up with it after failing to blow his brains out. I'll put you down for a kipper, shall I?'

41

'Oh, what the hell. I'll have the kedgeree anyway. I can always skip lunch, I suppose. Thank you.'

'And what about one of our lovely melons to start? Perfectly ripe honeydew. Sheer ambrosia. Virtually calorie free.'

'Yes, that does sound rather nice. I think I will. Thank you.'

'And you, sir?'

'I'll have a kipper, please, and half a grapefruit to start.'

'Why?' asked Sebastian. 'They're just sour oranges. Or big round lemons.'

'I read somewhere they suppress the appetite or something.'

'Of course they do. They're horrible.'

'Usual for Sebastian,' continued the landlord.

'What is your usual, Sebo?' I asked.

'Coffee,' he said quickly, with a glance at Robert.

'I'd like coffee too, please,' I said.

'And I'd like workman's tea, please. Very strong.'

'Another coffee and a strong pot of Indian tea coming up.' The publican pocketed his notebook, retrieved our menus and bustled off to the kitchen.

'Have you clicked who that is? By the door?' Sebastian asked.

'The hunched bald guy who looks like Bill Table the MP?' I asked. 'Who is he?'

'Bill Table the MP.'

'He looks miserable.'

'His wife's probably been getting at him again. You know she's leapfrogged him into the House of Lords? She was always the real politician, of course. He's just a very good-hearted, public-spirited man.'

'But hang on, *he* was the MP?'

'Yes, but she's got the real balls and drive – politically, anyway. She won and kept that seat for him. He just tagged along behind. And now she's completely eclipsed him in Parliament.'

'Well done them, though. They're a team,' said Reggie wistfully. 'They both earned that. Must be incredibly proud. Rather special to be made a lord.'

'But the whole thing's rigged, isn't it?' said Sebastian, surprised. 'Virtually meaningless: all down to brown envelopes and Buggins' turn. No real merit involved. Didn't Cameron make his hairdresser a dame or something?'

'Are you saying there's no real merit in hairdressing? I don't think George would agree. Would you, George?'

'A hell of a lot more merit than in head-hunting, that's for sure,' I admitted.

The publican came back over to clear the fourth place, the spare cutlery, plate and glass.

'So Wellington had nothing to do with Waterloo?' Reggie continued, becoming serious. 'Or Marlborough Blenheim? What about Maggie?'

'Should have been made a duchess,' interjected the landlord.

'Like Fergie,' said Sebastian sweetly.

'It must be depressing being so cynical, Sebo,' said Reggie. 'The Tables have worked their arses off for Britain. They deserve a bit of recognition. I'd be proud as anything.'

'I concede they do seem to do a lot, in and out of Parliament.'

'They're on telly non-stop: she trying to explain away the latest balls-up in the NHS, not an easy row to hoe, and he

43

beavering away for whichever London university he does that property thing for – one of those acronyms – for nothing as far as I can tell. Isn't he arch-steward-extraordinary or something?'

'Something like that. That's why I've been chatting him up: he has the final say on some of the most magnificent buildings in London; I'm rather hoping I might be able to give him a hand finding pictures for those acres of bare wall. I could use a decent new client, with the wedding coming up and maybe having to pay Spatchcock subs again.'

'Do you think he has anything to do with pitches and playing fields?'

'Very possibly.' Sebastian waved at the man who waved back.

'How did you meet him?' Reggie waved too.

'Bumpèd into him with Jerry at Christie's. Viewing that sporting auction.'

'Does he play cricket?' Reggie enquired innocently.

'I didn't ask,' Sebastian snapped. 'Hands off. He's mine.'

'All's fair in love and war,' said Reggie, waving again.

A waitress brought our coffee and tea and then returned with the porridge, grapefruit and melon. Sebastian carefully poured a lake of runny dark honey into the middle of his porridge, licking his lips, ringed it with a loop of cream, and picked up his spoon.

'Are you sure that's allowed?' Reggie bridled, pop-eyed with indignation.

'Absolutely.'

'That's not a diet. It's a feast! You're not dieting at all!'

'It's called the Fast Diet.'

'Fast Diet indeed!' spat Reggie, the sheer injustice sparking a jet of fury. 'How can it be fast, stuffing your face like that?'

'Not quick fast, break fast. You know, fasting. Not eating.'

'And you call that not eating?'

'You're such a communist, Reggie. If you can't have it, you can't bear anyone else having it.'

'Not at the moment, no!' Reggie agreed, scratching pitifully at his melon rind. 'But you're *not* fasting.'

'It doesn't *work* like that. You don't have to fast every day. Just two days a week. I can't believe you haven't heard of it: the Fast Diet? It's also called the Five Two. Two days a week fasting, and five days feasting, eating normally.'

'Yes, in your case eating normally *is* feasting.'

'Easy, tiger! You're the one obsessed with his paunch. This is your project. Don't get narky just because I'm managing it better than you are.'

'What do you mean "better"? I've lost sixteen pounds!'

'Water retention! And you started earlier!'

'But surely you can't eat anything? It doesn't stack up.'

'Literally anything and everything on the five non-fast days a week.'

'It's not fair! I've thrown out every cake, biscuit, crisp and chocolate in the house. Everything! All that cheese.'

'Me too, now the boys have gone back,' I agreed sadly. 'Even the nuts.'

'What a waste. Nothing to you fat cats, of course. But those of us with an artistic rather than commercial bent have to count our pennies.'

'But not your calories.' Reggie found the whole concept incomprehensible.

'Of course! But only on the two fast days. I'm not allowed more than six hundred calories on a fast day.'

'Six hundred? That's nothing.' After two weeks' dieting I could spot a calorie at thirty paces.

'Couldn't agree more. Yesterday I had a half-pint of madeira and a raw onion.'

'Yuk.'

'I'm fasting on Sundays and Wednesdays. Wednesdays are always busy, so they're hell, of course, but at least I'm distracted. Yesterday was agony. I managed to hang on till lunchtime. I gulped down the madeira at one and then crunched through the onion, by which time it was ten past, with no prospect of grub till the following morning – today, now – so I just did stuff, frantically, all day. I mucked out the whole flat. Found almost three quid in the sofa. Polished all my shoes, cleaned the windows. Even scraped out the oven. It was all I could do not to lick the gunk off the scraper. At nine I was so hungry I went to bed.'

'My heart aches,' said Reggie.

'Not half as much as my gut did.' Sebastian took a swig of coffee. 'I was gagging for that porridge.' He ran a pudgy finger round the inside of the empty bowl. 'Mmmmm. Wholesome.'

'So the fast days aren't consecutive?'

Sebastian took his finger out of his mouth. 'No, thank goodness. Not sure I could manage that. Though the inventor, or innovator, nice doctor with a lisp who promoted the whole idea,

46

seems to imply there are more health benefits if you do. Things like staving off dementia and diabetes.'

'Really?' Reggie was intrigued. 'I didn't know the two were linked.'

'Don't ask me. I was more interested in the mechanics than the medicine. Forgotten most of the rest. But it's how prehistoric man evolved to eat, apparently: kill a mammoth, gorge for five days, then take two days to find and dispatch another: probably bullshit, of course. The point is we're not doing this for health reasons, are we? You want to look svelte, Reggie, and George and I are just giving you moral support. Though George's wife might sleep a bit better if he wasn't such a tub of lard.'

'Coming from a man who hasn't seen his own dick in ten years . . .' I retorted, mildly.

'Who said I wanted to?'

'Touché,' said Reggie.

'Look. It's working for me: iron discipline for two days a week and then free as a bird on the others. What are you doing?'

'We're eating less,' Reggie replied through gritted teeth. 'Commonly known as dieting.'

'And you've done very well.' Sebastian poured himself another coffee. 'Though you don't look any different, except a hell of a lot glummer, but we can't deny the facts. The scales don't lie.'

'I'm still snoring, though,' I admitted. 'And struggling. Yesterday I ate a whole celery cluster – or bunch, or whatever you call it – and two cucumbers . . . in secret!'

'Two cucumbers? Pathetic.'

'While Fiona was watching *The X Factor*.'

'Why in secret? That's about two and a half calories. You were sticking to your diet.'

'I didn't want her to see me packing my face. It seemed ... it felt ... so greedy.'

'After twenty-five years, your greed'll probably come as the most awful surprise,' Reggie said.

'Though one shouldn't snack,' Sebastian chided primly. 'Everyone knows that.' The kitchen door slammed and he looked up like a questing Velociraptor. 'Is that the toast?' It wasn't. 'I hate celery.'

'So do I,' I said. 'Stringy with a rather unpleasant taste. I know it's spoilt, but this diet grub is so incredibly unsatisfying. And Fiona's such a brilliant cook it seems such a waste. Something's missing.'

'The x factor,' said Sebastian.

'Whatever it is, I go to bed feeling almost ripped off. I find myself lying in bed grinding my teeth and listening to my stomach gurgling.'

'What does Fiona prefer? Snoring, grinding or gurgling?' Sebastian asked.

'I've replaced food with water,' said Reggie. 'Glass after glass: about twelve a day.'

'Something polite to do with your lips,' said Sebastian.

'You must be peeing non-stop.'

'I was anyway.'

'Probably frightfully good for you,' I ventured, trying to be encouraging. 'We're all supposed to drink two litres a day, aren't we? Cleansing or something?'

'Bound to be,' Reggie replied bleakly. 'Detox.'

'You started this,' Sebastian pointed out, grinning and waving at a waitress carrying a toast rack just conceivably destined for us. 'No one's forcing you. If you don't like it, give up and save us all a thoroughly miserable four months. That's a whole third of a year! And according to current statistics, I only have twenty-four years left.'

'How are your candidates taking it? And your clients?' Reggie asked me, turning away from Sebastian. 'When you're forcing down the cucumbers like a sword swallower? And swatting away the chips?'

'Are you allowed mayonnaise? No point in chips without mayonnaise,' put in Sebastian.

'Your candidates don't resent you not joining in, George?' Reggie sighed, trying to ignore Sebastian. 'When you're wining and dining them? Don't feel you're being a party pooper?'

'Funnily enough, they don't seem to mind. They're being amazingly understanding and mellow. But I'm not being that draconian: I do trim the fat off meat . . .'

'Talk about wet,' scoffed Sebastian.

'. . . but mostly stick to fish or chicken, masses of greens and white wine or water, and avoid butter, sauces, puddings, liqueurs and cheese.'

'Cheese!' Reggie repeated softly, half closing his eyes.

'What?' said Sebastian. 'Speak up.'

'Cheese is just a memory,' Reggie whimpered, biting his hand. He was a leading light in the Worshipful Company of Cheesemongers.

The waitress set a rack of half-slices of white toast on the table, poured us more coffee and tea and cleared away our bowls and plates. Sebastian broke a piece of toast into fragments and buried one under a slab of white butter.

'Unsalted,' he explained, as if that made it any better, and then heaped it with great gloops of chunky black marmalade. He raised it to his mouth, noticed our horrified expressions and burst out laughing before he could eat it.

'Do cheer up,' he said, trying again.

'But it's so unfair!' said Reggie, wrenching his gaze from the toast. 'And nonsensical!' Sebastian managed to get the toast into his mouth before starting to laugh through the crumbs. 'You can't eat jam! It's crazy!'

'I can eat what I like ... on the Fast Diet. Anyway, marmalade's not jam; technically it's jelly, with the pulp left in,' Sebastian said officiously. 'Or in this case not pulp, but great bitter chunks of black rind. Mmmm. And it's medicinal. Mary Queen of Scots and Marie Antoinette swore by it for headaches, hence "*Marie est malade*", until the executioner came up with a more permanent ... answer.'

The landlord arrived with our plates, one containing a kipper, one the kedgeree, and the last piled with scrambled eggs, bacon, black pudding, fried bread, sausages and chips. The waitress placed mustard, mayonnaise, ketchup, brown sauce and what appeared to be a small vase of oil floating on petrol at Sebastian's elbow. Reggie's eyebrows shot through the roof.

'Black velvet,' said the publican. 'Mr Grace Brown's usual. Fifty-fifty Guinness and champagne, with the Guinness added

50

last over a spoon to keep the two separate. House speciality. Named after the velvet lining of Prince Albert's coffin. Lovely.'

'Perfect pick-me-up,' Sebastian assured us conspiratorially. 'Can I tempt you? You were both so tight-lipped and earnest earlier, I didn't dare suggest it.' He gingerly took a sip. 'Aaaah.'

Reggie flipped. 'Of course you can't tempt me!' he snapped, when the waitress and publican had fossicked off elsewhere. 'I'm on a fucking diet! I don't have alcohol at breakfast. I hardly have alcohol at all. It's a sugar. I have soft drinks because I'm trying to lose weight.'

'We don't need soft drinks.' Sebastian gestured towards the teapot with the heel of his glass. 'We're English. We have tea.'

'You don't even like tea.'

'I *love* tea, with sugar, lots of sugar, the idea of tea.'

'But you prefer Guinness and champagne?'

'Only on high days and holidays. It's bloody expensive, for a start. Normally I have coffee. Not champagne maybe, but certainly a cut above soft. Did you know the word coffee is in fact derived from the Arab word for wine, *qahwah*.'

'No.'

'And rather like wine, which is integral to so many religions, coffee roasting, grinding and brewing were first recorded in the Sufi shrines of fifteenth-century Yemen.'

'And then it was taken up by all those Sufi shrines in England?'

'It spread from Africa to Persia to Turkey to Europe, hitting London in the 1650s. And every coffee house had its own character. Those interested in shipping went to Lloyd's coffee house, which became the centre of global insurance. Those interested in stocks and shares went to Jonathan's, which became the Stock Exchange. And those with no interests whatsoever went to the dear old Spatchcock.'

'You are the master of red herrings, Sebo. I give up.'

'Talking of herrings,' I said, piercing a bronze shard with my fork and putting it in my mouth. 'I haven't had kippers in years.' I grimaced. 'Now I remember why.' I swallowed it anyway.

'Those are the best kippers in Britain,' said Sebastian, confounded by my wincing and mumbling.

'But they're still kippers,' I said blankly, having forced it down.

'I love kippers,' said Sebastian reproachfully.

'Well, why aren't you having them then?'

'I never have fish before lunch,' he said, picking up his knife and fork. 'Unless I've caught it myself.'

Reggie had finished his kedgeree, and I was struggling with my kipper, and neither of us could help watching Sebastian with real resentment.

His four slices of streaky bacon were golden crisp and yet thick enough to retain a sweaty, unctuous quality. The scrambled egg was bright orange with butter and organic yolk, and the black pudding was a damp purple-brown. Sebastian brushed a morsel of black pudding on to a gold-frosted splinter of fried bread and topped it with a smear of egg, before wedging in a flake of bacon. He raised his fork, steadied the agglomeration for a moment, and then ate it.

I realised my mouth was open . . . and shut it.

'That's neat fat!' Reggie blasted, genuinely aggrieved.

52

'Yes, I miss it on fast days.' Sebastian took another slug of black velvet. 'It's delicious and terribly good for you.'

'Don't lecture me about fat, Sebo. Or cholesterol. I know it all.'

'Is it fat or cholesterol that causes high blood pressure?' I asked.

'High blood pressure is caused by cholesterol, George, which comes from fat.'

'Actually, I think you'll find that's all nonsense.'

'They have now identified good and bad fats and good and bad cholesterol,' Reggie ploughed on.

'They keep changing their minds,' Sebo said. 'They'll change back again soon. Whichever was good is bad and whichever was bad is good. It's all meaningless.'

'Saturated with what?' I asked. 'Types of fat?'

Sebastian pinned another lump of black pudding onto a fragment of fried bread and levered it into his mouth. He looked up at Reggie, crunched a few times and swallowed. 'Come on then, fat expert. What the hell does it mean?'

'Okay.' Reggie frowned with concentration. 'Unsaturated fat comes from vegetable, nut and fish oil and is generally regarded as good. Saturated fat, which is normally solid and white at room temperature, is from animals.'

'Ah, creeping vegetarianism. Of course. Humans who eat animals are bad humans. Everyone must eat bark and grass to keep them weak and feeble so they do what the nice eco-wankers tell them to.'

'Nothing to do with vegetarianism, Sebo. Saturated fat doesn't just come from animals, it's in coconut and palm oil too, and it does have higher levels of cholesterol, but now they think it's not the *amount* of cholesterol but the *type*: good or bad.'

'Moving the bloody goalposts again.'

'The real baddies seem to be "trans fats", the synthetic stuff they add to fast and processed food.'

'Why do they add this stuff to food, Reggie? If it's so poisonous?' I asked.

'Texture and shelf life. And of course they didn't know it was bad for you originally; just trying to get people fed. But it turns out that trans fats are sodden with low-density lipids, which is bad cholesterol.'

'What's good cholesterol then?'

'High-density lipids, which actually protect the heart.'

'You really have done your research, Reggie,' said Sebastian, looking up from his plate again.

'I'm taking it seriously,' said Reggie, pouring himself another cup of tea. 'Unlike some of us.'

'We all are,' Sebastian insisted, wiping his mouth on his napkin with a slightly aggrieved air and pushing his plate away. 'That was bliss. Unutterable bliss: kedgeree, kippers, eggs, bacon, fried bread, black pudding, sausages and chips all brought to perfection at exactly the same time and placed piping hot in front of us, just when we want it. Stupendous.'

I gave up on my kipper, having exposed the skin from the inside, one of the most revolting meals I'd had in a very long time, and gurned at Sebastian.

'It occurred to me,' Sebastian continued, 'that timing is very important in this dieting business.'

54

'Timing is important,' Reggie agreed cautiously, still feeling rather empty despite the kedgeree. 'It seems that some scientists now recommend eating only in the hours of daylight, for instance.'

'I don't understand,' Sebastian said.

'In pre-history, Stone Age man only ate in daylight.'

'Really? Doesn't sound very likely.' I was feeling empty too. 'What about all that feasting round the communal fire and sharing boar carcasses or whatever? With wolves howling just beyond the light and children fighting over the bones?'

'Never happened,' said Reggie.

'Don't believe you,' I said.

'Okay, maybe it happened,' conceded Reggie, 'but we'd evolved into what we are before then, before we discovered fire. No one eats in the dark, do they, by choice? Before fire we had to eat in daylight and that's what our bodies evolved to do.'

'I thought we were only able to evolve big brains after we'd learnt to get more energy from our food by cooking it? Which required fire,' Sebastian said.

'And actually,' I said rather smugly, having read an article on this very topic on Sunday, 'recent research suggests that eating in the dark, or wearing a blindfold, cons you into thinking you've eaten more, so you eat less.'

'Well, that wasn't a problem in the Stone Age, was it? Eating too much?' Sebastian insisted. 'They were all on the bloody Atkins without even realising it, weren't they? Or the Fast Diet? Whoever heard of Stone Age men "watching what they ate"? They were far too worried about being eaten themselves! And that's not what I meant, anyway. I was talking about when we weigh ourselves. All the books and articles I've looked at say you should weigh yourself once a week, not once a fortnight, and very first thing in the morning.'

'I actually weigh myself every day, as soon as I get up,' I said. 'After a pee, before a coffee, before even putting the dogs out, stark bollock naked and trying not to touch the wall. I've got brand-new scales.'

'Do you? Have you?' Now Sebastian looked really aggrieved. 'That's a bit sneaky.'

'No it isn't. I like to see exactly how much more I have to go to keep myself on the straight and narrow.'

'So what are we doing at the Spatchcock? Why are we bothering with this fortnightly farce?'

'We've only done it twice. What do you mean farce?'

'I mean futile waste of time. I mean hollow formality. What is the point of solemnly meeting in London once a fortnight if you're furtively weighing yourself anyway every day at home?'

'I've bought myself scales too, Sebo,' Reggie admitted.

'Why?'

'To see how I'm doing. There's nothing furtive about it.'

'Well I'm a bit . . . pissed off. It's cheating.'

'Look,' Reggie poured Sebastian some more coffee and passed him the milk. 'There's no such thing as cheating as far as our diet's concerned. It's not a competition. We have the same goal and we're trying to help each other get there.'

'Well . . .'

'I only suggested fortnightly because you both have proper jobs and I assumed you couldn't manage any more,' Reggie explained. 'Of course you're absolutely right about the time of day, but we're all eating so little I don't think it really matters if it's first thing or lunchtime.'

He watched as Sebastian took another draught of black velvet and licked the foam from his upper lip. 'Most of us anyway.'

'When's our next meeting?' asked Sebastian.

'We're all shooting in Essex on the last Saturday in January, aren't we? Just before Jane and I go away. Why don't we meet on the Friday?'

'Perfect,' I replied. 'My turn to cough up. We'll meet at the Spatchcock at twelve thirty for our weigh-in and I'll book that new restaurant behind Regent Street for one: Mintons. Apparently their fish is unbelievable.'

'What about their chips?' Sebastian jeered, raising his glass again and winking at Reggie. 'And mayonnaise, of course?'

CHAPTER 3

'Buy at the sound of gunfire. Sell at the sound of trumpets.'

Old Stock Exchange adage

Sebastian took over his uncle's shoot syndicate ten years ago. Though the costs are shared, Sebastian is very much in charge and deals with the landowners, the gamekeeper, the members and the money, in exchange for free membership himself. The members – 'guns' – and the beaters gather at his uncle's old house before each shoot, as they have always done, and his aunt, Fleur, still presides over lunch and tea. Sebastian snaffled Reggie for the syndicate the minute he arrived in Essex and, being such close neighbours and friends, either or both ask me to shoot every year.

Since his divorce and her widowhood, Sebastian makes a point of burning up the A12 on his motorbike at least twice a month to visit his aunt, bringing chocolates for her and her housekeeper, Pam, and normally staying the night.

For various reasons we had been unable to make our planned weigh-in on the Friday, but as I was shooting with the syndicate as Reggie's guest on the Saturday, we decided to do the deed on his new scales in the kitchen before the shoot.

Jane dropped us off in the stable yard at nine. We left our gear at the back door with the dogs and took our guns and Reggie's scales inside.

We walked straight through to the kitchen and found Sebastian preparing elevenses. He was wearing a shirt and tie, thick jersey, tweed britches and long woolly shooting socks, and fussing over a collection of baskets, boxes and Thermos flasks.

'Morning, Sebo,' hissed Reggie in a stage whisper, symbolic recognition that Sebastian's aunt should not be disturbed.

'Reggie. George,' Sebastian replied tensely. He was always edgy before a shoot. 'Coffee?' He waved at the kettle.

'Let's get the weighing over first, shall we?' said Reggie, placing the dark plastic scales in the centre of the floor. He pressed the edge a couple of times with his toe to check it was level, triggering the appearance of a string of bright green zeros. Then flattened our page out on the kitchen table.

'I don't think I've lost a bean,' said Sebastian mournfully.

'Of course you have, Sebo,' said Reggie, stepping back to look at him. 'Hard to tell in jersey and britches. Five or six pounds, I should think?'

'But only on the wrists and cock,' said Sebastian. 'All I needed.'

'I'll go first then, shall I?' Reggie offered, and not waiting for an answer pulled his own jersey over his head, kicked off his shoes, patted his flanks to check there was nothing in his pockets, and stepped on the scales.

The bright green zeros flickered to 15:13.

'Another five pounds!' I said. 'And I was clapping *myself* on the back.'

'Slowing down,' harrumphed Sebastian, ungenerously.

'To be expected,' Reggie replied. 'Your turn.'

'Just got to mix this soup. Let George go first.' He emptied a carton of tomato juice into a steaming saucepan of beef consommé, and then added Tabasco and Worcestershire sauce and salt and pepper, stirring carefully with a wooden spoon and sipping occasionally. 'Won't be a minute.'

I had lost three and a half pounds. 'Not bad,' said Sebastian, tightening the lid on a Thermos flask. He noticed my belt. 'Though these scales and the Spatchcock's will be completely out of sync. What belt hole are you on now?'

'Six,' I admitted coyly. 'Down from eight.'

'Progress at any rate,' he conceded, hauling off his jersey and kicking his shoes away. 'My turn.'

'Oh, bloody hell!' he fumed, teetering into a squat with a whine of flatulence as he tried to get as close as possible to the reading. He touched the floor, coughed, farted again and fell off. 'I told you! I've actually *gained* a fucking pound!' He stood up. 'It's these ridiculous sodding scales.'

'Or breakfast?' said Reggie, eyeing a dirty pan in the sink. Sebastian got back on the scales again, scowled and got off.

'Bugger.'

'So much for the *Fast* Diet,' Reggie goaded. He had not forgotten the Cock and Bull. 'I knew you couldn't eat just anything.'

'You bloody well can!'

'Sometimes a cup of coffee can add a pound, Sebo,' I said. 'I always weigh myself before I've had anything, even water.'

'Oh, well done you, George! Thanks for the tip! It's hardly progress, though, is it? Even without that extra "coffee pound"?' He jammed a bottle of sloe gin home with a creak of wicker and a high-pitched clink. 'Four whole days in the last fortnight eating like Twiggy – not just agony but bloody boring – and I *put on* weight. It's ludicrous.'

'When's your next fast day?'

'Tomorrow. If I bother.' He took a tray of sausage rolls out of the oven, wrapped them in silver foil and then a tea towel and slid the hot bundle into an insulated Danger Mouse lunch box. 'Would you mind helping me put all this crap on the wagon?'

We put our shoes and jerseys back on and Reggie and I carried our guns and the boxes and baskets out through the gun room to the stable yard.

The cobbled square was ringed with brick buildings, the house on one side, stables and coach house on the others, and entered from the road through a large arch, topped by a blue-faced clock.

There was plenty of room for the cars and the gun wagon, a covered trailer with facing benches pulled by a Land Rover, to wait in front of the coach house. The beaters' wagon, much bigger and towed by a tractor, drew up on the verge outside.

Having finished briefing the twenty or thirty beaters and picker-uppers, and having dished out the flags and walkie-talkies, Brian the gamekeeper came over to give us a hand with the baskets. Sebastian emerged from the house with his gun, coat, cartridge bag and hat, hurriedly stowed them in the back of the gun wagon and popped back out again to greet the beaters. Then he led us into the coach house.

There no longer being a coach, or even a pony, a wood burner had been installed in the coach house and a kitchen plumbed into the tack room next door. Brian's wife June was clearing away the beaters' empty mugs and preparing to lay the trestle tables for their lunch. The guns eat with Sebastian's Aunt Fleur in the hall.

We poured ourselves coffee while Sebastian theatrically shuffled the game cards, and the scrunch of tyres on the cobbles outside signalled the arrival of more guns.

Brian sounded his horn, calling the beaters to the tractor and trailer. Sebastian slung more logs in the wood burner and Reggie picked up the cards.

'Who else have we got today?' he asked, turning to the list of guns on the back of the cards. 'I did tell you I'd invited a woman along? Just to watch. A rather glorious Yank.'

'Yes,' nodded Sebastian. 'Something to do with the Dolls' House Trust?' For various reasons to do with his wealth, charm and 'portable building expertise', Reggie had been bamboozled into becoming chairman of the Dolls' House Trust, a sort of National Trust for dolls' houses, and is now the darling of every little girl in England, whatever her age.

'Yes. She's just given us the most enormous donation and wanted to see a shoot. She also wants to "share some ideas" about giving the trust "more reach".'

'That sounds ominous. Like what?' Reggie had cajoled Sebastian into becoming the trust art director – unpaid, as Sebastian never let us forget.

'Offering reproductions of some of the dolls' houses on her shopping channel, and giving the trust a big slice of the profits.'

'Well, make sure it's a big slice of the proceeds, Reggie, regardless of profits. Get the formula carved in stone. They should take all the risk. We're a charity, not a business. And they should be made, "reproduced", if at all possible, in England, preferably Essex.'

'The lawyers can sort all that if and when it comes to it, but you will be kind to her today won't you, Sebo? Please? She's our guest . . . and I like the idea of getting the collection out there.'

'They don't call me bird magnet for nothing, Reggie, but *you* can bring her back when she gets cold feet, literally or mentally. Have you got her a shooting stick and earmuffs?'

'No. Good idea. But it's only for the morning. She's got to get straight back after lunch.' Reggie looked round to see if Pam was about. 'What are we having?'

'Venison. Our very own muntjac and mash.'

'Delicious.' Reggie rubbed his hands and then froze. 'I've just had a thought. What if she's a vegetarian?'

'She can have cereal.'

'No, I mean it.'

'She's hardly likely to ask to see a shoot if she's a rabid vegan, is she? Stop panicking.'

'Good point.'

64

'And you asked the colonel!' Sebastian exclaimed. 'Why? Impossible old git. I preferred him when he was fat.'

'He's not that bad. One of the few Spatchcock members prepared to take on the new chairman, for one thing. Actually gnashes his teeth and froths at the mouth. Anyway, Damian pulled out at the last minute: work crisis.' Damian is one of Reggie's sons-in-law. 'Weren't many other takers at one day's notice.'

'Ah.'

I looked over Reggie's shoulder at the list of guns.

'So the colonel does have a Christian name.'

'Two Christian names,' said Sebastian.

'I never took him for a Valentine.'

A brutally ugly and overweight ginger mongrel hobbled into the room, followed by its nattily dressed and equally overweight master and the other dogs and guns. Minute, immaculate and huffily apologetic, the colonel arrived last, having got lost.

When everyone who wanted it had coffee or tea, Sebastian invited us each to pick a game card from the fan in his hand, a number on the underside of each card determining our peg on the first drive. He gave us a brief pep talk and safety lecture and we filtered back outside.

A dark blue Bentley rolled into the yard and pulled up next to the gun wagon. The driver handed a woman out of the car. She was in her forties, perhaps, and dressed in eighteen-hole Doc Marten boots of the same bright red as her lipstick, leather trousers, and an upholstered coat with a fur-trimmed hood. She had a Great Gatsby-type bob, hair very black against her white skin and teeth, and a round face, despite her slim build, made even rounder by a fixed smile as Reggie introduced us one by one.

'Shandy Madison,' she said. 'Founder and president of the English Channel. Thank you for having me today.'

'The what?' asked Sebastian.

'The English Channel,' Reggie explained hurriedly. 'The television channel in America. Specialising in all things English. Shandy's the founder, the president and the star.'

'Oh, of course,' said Sebastian.

'Never heard of it,' said the colonel. Reggie quickly helped him into the gun wagon.

The driver took a thick bundle of gladioli from the back of the Bentley.

'For our hostess,' Shandy explained.

'Oh, you mean my aunt?' Sebastian replied, taking a second to twig. 'I'm not sure she's ready to see anyone quite yet. But she'll love them, of course.' He took the flowers. 'Ah June,' he hailed the gamekeeper's wife. 'Can you look after these till we get back, please?'

'My car returns at quarter of two. Does that work with you guys?' Shandy asked.

'Perfect,' said Sebastian.

The rest of us piled into the gun wagon and we set off.

It was a lovely morning, though quite cold in the wind, with high white clouds churning across the vast Essex sky. My two dogs and I were number eight on the first drive, at the upper left-hand end of a horseshoe of guns below a strip of maize, our backs to the river. A hedge ran down the right-hand edge of the maize and then continued on down, dividing the field and bisecting the line of guns, who were spread out to my right at 35-yard intervals.

Tommy Styles, Fleur Grace Brown's stockbroker, looked particularly natty in his belted tweed Norfolk jacket and britches, long lavender socks, ankle boots, bow tie and fedora. He was twice the size Reggie had ever been and an inveterate dandy. From this distance his dog, Mikey, the beige mongrel, looked like a space hopper, an inflated rubber ball with a tiny face and ridged ear-handles that my boys had bounced around on when they were little. Tommy too looked almost spherical. Standing with Reggie, Shandy took their photograph on her telephone.

The beaters converged at the top of the strip of maize, sweeping in from the surrounding fields. Two passed me, flags held high, and pigeons began abandoning the trees in the hedge. A lone cock pheasant took to the air, crowing defiance, rising and rising. He set course for the river, impossibly high. His head went back, his wings folded and I heard the crack of Sebastian's 28-bore. A superb shot. A distant cheer came from the beaters above.

A partridge skimmed over from the right, more pheasants rocketed from the maize, and shots began popping along the line. The picker-uppers far behind – Dave with his four show Labradors, sleek as otters, Kevin with his springers, Sharon with her flat-coats, and Lady Barbara with her golden retriever and Jack Russell – sent dogs racing for the downed birds; all except the Jack Russell, hysterically straining against her reinforced harness, yearning and yapping with manic glee.

At the end of the drive, the beaters and their dogs walked on through the pegs, picking up any missed fallen birds and congratulating or commiserating with the guns. A cock pheasant had been left in the plough for the ancient mongrel Mikey, who waddled unsteadily past it until Tommy scooped him up and, cradling him in his arms and grunting with the effort, bent down until the dog's pug-like muzzle was almost resting on the bronze plumage. Drooling, Mikey opened his foam-flecked jaws and grasped the pheasant. Applause broke out again and his master carried the pair off in triumph.

After the second drive we paused for elevenses. The beater and gun wagons were parked in the lee of a wood. A great lover of kit, Sebastian was proud of his picnic paraphernalia, which he spread out on a folding table.

There were two wicker bottle baskets containing sloe gin, cherry brandy, damson vodka, ginger liqueur, cava, white burgundy and sherry, and Thermos flasks of soup, tea, coffee and milk. There were the sausage rolls and diagonally striped triangles of hot *croque monsieur* in a Clangers freezer bag. He flung back the lid of a small trunk packed with biscuits, chocolates, apples, tangerines, paper napkins, shatterproof globular glasses, little bottles of water, cans of soft drink, lager, mugs and two or three corkscrews.

Having made sure everyone who wanted it had soup, Sebastian began mixing sloe-gasms – sloe gin and cava – and Tommy dished them out. Seeing Reggie and me empty handed, he held out two glasses.

'I'm driving,' we chimed in unison, rather too hastily.

'I thought Jane was collecting you?' said Tommy. 'I was promised a seat next to her at lunch.' Reggie blew his nose. Tommy offered the colonel a glass. 'Sloe-gasm, Val?' No one called him Val. He accepted the drink with a grunt.

'So it's true,' said Jerry, a semi-retired insurance broker, amateur pig breeder, and musterer of corporate support for Reggie's cricket charity. 'You really are dieting. And off the sauce too. I'd heard rumours of course. You don't have diabetes or anything?'

'Doesn't everyone?' quipped Sebastian, teeth clenched as he pulled a cork.

'No they do not,' barked the colonel, vexed by his own ineptitude all morning and Sebastian's phenomenal accuracy. As if in reply, *bang*: the cork came out with a noise like a shot.

'Why didn't you ask me? Nothing I don't know about dieting,' said Tommy. 'Been on a diet all my life.'

'The wrong one,' said the colonel.

'Not one, Val, many,' Tommy replied blithely, downing his own sloe-gasm. 'I'm what they call a yoyo dieter, but each time the string gets that little bit longer.' He selected a triangle of *croque monsieur*.

'Amazed it hasn't snapped,' said the colonel, fizzing with hostility. Tommy turned his broad back on him.

'Was it a New Year's thing, Sebo?' he asked. 'How's it actually going?'

'A Reggie thing,' Sebastian replied. 'Piece of cake. No trouble at all.'

'No progress at all,' growled the colonel, circumnavigating Tommy to get at the lunch box. 'In your case. But Lambert's lost weight.' He jabbed a sausage roll at Reggie. 'Your collar's loose.'

'I've come to the conclusion that it's not the choice of diet, but sticking to it that's the problem. I have lost weight but not my appetite so it has *not* been a piece of cake. Nor is it going to be sloe gin and sausage rolls either, thank you, Sebo. Though blimey I'm tempted.'

'Amazing the power of vanity,' said Sebastian, ostentatiously chomping on a second sausage roll.

'And greed,' huffed the colonel. 'You and ...' He pulled his game card out of his pocket and squinted at the list of guns on the back, and then at me. 'You and Courtauld haven't lost an ounce.'

'I wouldn't be rude to George, Valentine,' threatened Sebastian. 'He'll put you in one of his books.'

'Rude?' queried the colonel with genuine incredulity, before dismissing the idea as absurd. He stepped closer and peered up at me. 'Are you an author?'

'Publisher too,' said Sebastian.

'Even better,' said the colonel.

'He published his first book himself, and sold 140,000 copies in two weeks. Got to number six in the bestseller lists.'

'Well, you're in luck.' The colonel's beady gaze was unwavering. 'I have a manuscript for you: exceptional.'

'What's it about?' I asked.

'A remarkable spring and summer fifty years ago,' he replied.

'What's it called?' asked Jerry.

'It's All About Me Me,' said the colonel.

'That's the title?'

'Yes.'

'The thing is I'm ... I'm not really a proper publisher,' I explained.

'Not even for you you,' said Sebastian.

'I only ended up publishing my first book because no one else would. It was basically a one-off fluke. Just a list really.'

'Well here's your chance to *become* a proper publisher, if proper means profitable.'

'Valentine?' said Reggie, gamely trying to rescue me, 'is that yours?' A padded gun-sleeve of fresh pink hide was leaning against the nearest tractor wheel.

'What? The gun-sleeve? No, mine's canvas,' the colonel replied sharply, riled at the interruption. 'I'm talking to George, Lambert.'

'Mine,' said Jerry. 'Christmas present to myself. Boris, my heroic old boar. Wanted something a bit more interactive than just a headstone after all those years of sterling service.'

'Remind me never to work for you, Jerry,' said Tommy.

'Pigskin,' said Sebastian, crestfallen. 'How very disappointing.' He forlornly helped himself to the last *croque monsieur*. 'Can nothing be relied on these days?'

'Your gluttony at least, Brown,' said the colonel, turning back to me. 'Now, about my book . . .'

'Talking of lists and books,' Reggie said hurriedly, still trying to distract the colonel and turning to Shandy, 'has Sebo told you about the list he's compiling for his granddaughter?' He beckoned at me. 'George? Colonel? You must listen to this.'

71

'She's due in July,' Sebo told them.

'Never too early to start,' said Shandy.

'Exactly,' said Sebastian. 'Books were the primary treat of my childhood; sort of gaming, films and computers all rolled into one, and a way of teleporting oneself away from all that unutterable boredom: interminable journeys; endless tagging along to grown-up stuff on best behaviour. I'll never forget the day I was given an entire set of Dickens, in miniature, with its own special mini-lockable rack and magnifying glass.'

'Drivel,' said the colonel. 'Claptrap.'

'That rack and a torch kept me happy for months,' Sebastian continued unabashed. 'And then one day I was allocated a real bookcase all of my own, with adjustable shelves.'

'What joy!' the colonel snorted. 'Where were you brought up? Wormwood Scrubs?'

'I spent hours arranging my books: by size or colour, like my crayons, or date or subject, even author.'

'What a tick,' said the colonel.

'What's first?' I asked. 'On your list?'

'*Jeremy Fisher*,' Sebastian replied. 'Always loved the newt's waistcoat.'

'Beatrix Potter does very well for us,' said Shandy.

'You sell books?' The colonel sidled closer, suddenly interested. 'Do you publish too?'

But Sebastian had not finished.

'*Ferdinand the Bull*, of course, *Stig of the Dump*. I'm rereading a lot at the moment to check they're as good as I remember. *The Call of the Wild*: heartbreaking. And *The Selfish Giant*.'

72

'Any not as good as you remember?' asked Tommy.

'Yes. *Robinson Crusoe*'s a bit stilted for a modern child, I think. Though I fantasised endlessly about having my own desert island.'

'She'll be branded a freak, Sebo, your poor granddaughter, when she starts school,' said Jeremy. 'For having read all that fuddy-duddy rubbish. For goodness' sake don't saddle her with your bonkers baggage!'

'Of course, Jerry, you're absolutely right. I won't bother. I'll let her be saddled with someone else's bonkers baggage.'

'I loved *Charlotte's Web*,' Shandy said.

'*Brilliant* idea, Shandy.' Sebastian whipped out a red notebook and scrawled something across a page.

'I've always liked female heroes,' Shandy said.

'Heroines,' said the colonel.

'What you really ought to read, Shandy,' Reggie said, 'if you like heroines, is Charles Moore's biography of Mrs T. I read the first volume on holiday last year. Cried like a baby. Taking the second one to Thailand next week. Can't wait.'

Shandy forced a smile.

'You haven't got a drink,' said Sebastian.

'I'm not thirsty.'

'Neither are we.' Sebastian poured them both a sloe-gasm.

She took a cautious sip and winced. 'What is it?'

'Sloe gin and cava.'

'Too mean for champagne, eh, Brown?'

'Yes, why don't we have champagne?' asked Jerry.

'No point mixing anything expensive with sloe gin.'

'Don't make the mistake of thinking inexpensive means inferior,' Shandy said. 'Cava's delicious, I'll have it without the gin please, Sebastian, and an awe-inspiring story.'

'What story?'

'The Spanish vines were hit by the phylloxera louse in the 1860s, virtually wiping them out.'

'The same plague that destroyed the vines in France and Italy?'

'It was global. But the vintners of Catalonia had mighty cojones. They looked around and followed the money. England was the richest country on earth back then, and a great consumer of champagne.'

'Still is, I think.'

'You're right. The Americans are now the biggest consumers by total value, but the English still lead the field by volume.'

'Good old us.'

'So the Catalonians decided to take on champagne. Tackle it head on, without all the time-consuming inefficiency and nonsensical traditions that make champagne so expensive.'

'I rather like all that,' said Sebastian.

'They replanted with white grapes, streamlined and mechanised as much of the process as they could, and opened the first cellars or "*cavas*" in the mid-1890s.'

'So *cava* means cellar? Like cave I suppose,' said Sebastian.

'I was lucky enough to be shown round by the great-grandson of one of the founders last year, part of a group thinking of replicating the success of the English Channel in Spain. The rest is history.'

'And that's why it's so much cheaper. I had no idea,' said Tommy, draining his second sloe-gasm. 'I'll try it neat too, then Sebo.'

'What about Prosecco?'

'Now Prosecco I do know about,' said Jerry. 'Read it in the cocktail menu in Harry's Bar on my honeymoon. Pliny, the chap who said "*in vino veritas*", the Ancient Roman, adored Prosecco.'

'Is it really that old?' said Reggie. 'You amaze me. Are you sure it isn't a made-up name? Always assumed it was some sort of marketeer's gimmick, like Babycham or Nutrasweet. I thought it was a play on *secco*: sort of "Go dry!"'

'It's a village near Venice.'

'So why were they writing about it in a cocktail menu?'

'Bellinis, of course. The cocktail: Prosecco and peach nectar. Invented in Harry's Bar before the war. Prosecco being local to Venice, and the cocktail itself being the same colour as the saint's toga.'

'What saint's toga?'

'The toga of a saint in a painting by Bellini in the church next door.'

'Well I never,' said Reggie.

'So we're sticking with cava then?' Sebastian laughed, holding out the bottle. The colonel cleared his throat behind me. My resolve crumpled.

'A glass of real wine for me, please, Sebastian. White. Thanks. To help my eye in.' I helped myself to a glass and filled it to the top. 'Just one.'

'Alcohol?' Shandy asked, wide-eyed with mock horror. 'And you say you're dieting?'

'Depends on the calories. I try to limit myself to two glasses of wine a day. I was going to have them both at lunch . . .'

'No battle plan survives first contact with the enemy,' said the colonel, sagely, gripping my elbow. 'Now about this manuscript, George.'

'Where are we off to next, Sebo?' I asked desperately.

It was twelve forty-five by the time we returned to the hall for lunch. Some of us dumped our clobber in the cars, and swapped boots for shoes. Tommy bowed over the bonnet of his Range Rover trying to pull a boot off, heaving and grunting, the thick neoprene heel in the grip of a crude wooden boot jack, a plank with a V cut in it resting on a cross bar. He writhed and jerked like a hooked fish, unable to pull out his foot.

'Too many sausages,' said Jerry. 'My sausages.'

'Fat feet,' said the colonel.

'Are you okay?' asked Shandy.

'This bloody boot jack,' puffed Tommy.

'It's very unusual.'

'Bloody unusual. It cost a hundred and thirty-five grand!' He heaved again.

'You're kidding! What's it made of? Rhinoceros horn?'

'I sent my son to one of the most expensive schools in England. Ugh! Ahh!' He yanked at his boot again. 'And after five long years, this is all either of us have to show for it.' As if inflamed by the thought he started stomping round the yard, boot jack

76

sticking out from his heel like a giant spur, banging and stamping. The jack squeaked, cracked and split, suddenly reduced to kindling, and everybody froze, until Tommy gathered up the pieces one by one and put them in his car.

We took our guns into the gun room just in time to stop Mikey from drinking from the downstairs loo, the water having turned a lurid blue, washed our hands and moved on into the hall.

Looking flushed and expectant in a violet wool dress, Fleur Grace Brown, Sebastian's aunt, was waiting in a wingchair by the hall fire, next to a tray of tiny glasses and a decanter of sherry. A disordered *Times* lay on the ottoman in front of her. The sherry glasses were so small I felt only a spasm of remorse as I helped everyone to a glass, including myself; everyone except Reggie, who was sticking to fizzy water.

'Nothing tastes as good as looking this good feels,' he said, adding ice and lemon to his San Pellegrino.

'It jolly well does,' said Tommy.

'Successful morning?' Fleur enquired.

'Good, thank you.' Sebastian replied. 'But what's happened to the gun-room loo? The water's gone funny. Mikey nearly died.'

'Lead shot; wouldn't flush away. I promised Pam you'd deal with it, but you never did. She has her professional pride, knew Reggie was bringing a special guest (an American for goodness' sake, light years ahead of us in the loo department), so she perfectly reasonably tried to mask it in the meanwhile with some sort of coloured cleaning liquid. I'd forgotten about the dogs.'

'I warned her about the pheasant casseroles,' said Sebastian. 'Where's the toasting fork? And I'll need some candle stubs.'

He snatched the three-pronged toasting fork from the fireplace and trotted back to the gun room. Fleur shuddered, then saw Reggie.

'Tell me it's not true,' she shouted from her chair, in a voice that could spark class war at thirty paces. 'You're a positive husk. Tell me you're not doing a marathon.'

'Of course I'm not, Fleur,' Reggie replied, walking over. 'Absolute twaddle. I'm just easing back on the grub for a few months.' He bent to kiss her. 'Gluttony-lite.'

'I am relieved. Nothing worse than over-exertion at our age.' She was at least ten years older than Reggie.

'Have you met my guest? The girl in the dashing leather trousers: Shandy Madison.'

'Shandy? Is that an actual name?'

'She's American. The American I told you about.'

'I love Americans and they adore me.'

'And Shandy's terrific. Been standing with me all morning: clever, feisty and fun. Just gone to fetch the flowers she brought you.'

'You think everyone's terrific, Reggie.'

'She's scouting for her television channel. I've asked her to the Cheesemongers' dinner.'

'You've never asked me to a Cheesemongers' dinner.'

'You don't like cheese.'

'But I love dressing up. I can't remember the last time I wore a tiara.' Slightly miffed, she turned as Shandy appeared and accepted her hand.

'Shandy Madison,' said Reggie. 'Fleur Grace Brown.'

78

'Thank you for having me in your lovely home, Mrs Grace Brown,' Shandy gushed. 'And yes, it *is* an actual name; short for Chanterelle.'

'The mushroom? How . . . unusual.'

'The treble string on a lute, actually,' Shandy insisted.

'Of course. Sh . . . Beautiful.' Fleur faltered. 'I shall just have to call you "darling". I'm Fleur.'

'Shandy,' said the colonel. 'Neither one thing nor the other.'

'These are for you, Fleur.' Shandy turned to Tommy, who had carried the heavy flowers through from the gun room for her and took them in her arms. She tried to lay the bolster of damp vegetation in her hostess's lap but Tommy helped Fleur deflect them on to the newspaper.

'I never get flowers any more. What a treat, but perhaps leave them on the ottoman just for now. Thank you. Have you had a good morning?'

'Awesome.'

'And how do you know Reggie?'

'The Dolls' House Trust,' Reggie explained. 'Shandy wants to introduce us to America.'

'Through the telly?'

'Yes. I'm president of the English Channel.'

'Wonderful. And English programmes? I gather the new Sherlock Holmes is very popular abroad?'

'What happened to Basil Brush?' demanded the colonel, who had tired of the miniature glasses and moved on to gin and tonic. 'And Doctor Who?'

'Doctor Who's still going strong. They're having a woman doctor next.'

'Not another fucking old Etonian.'

'We focus on retail,' Shandy explained. Fleur looked none the wiser.

'Shopping,' said Reggie.

'And you presumably pop over to England all the time?'

'This is my first visit actually, Fleur. My colleagues and I feel it's time we had a presence here. I expect to be in London regularly over the coming months.'

'Though she does know Spain,' said Reggie.

'Well then, you can't refuse my delicious sherry; a very special dry Oloroso. It's *so* good I tantalise everyone with these miniature glasses. The only chance I get to use them.'

'They are tiny,' Shandy laughed, picking one up and holding it against the light. 'And such delicate engraving.'

'Completely out of fashion now, of course, and totally worthless, but they're actually late eighteenth century.'

'Something Jane Austen's Emma might have used, or Mr Darcy.'

'We had the "tax on light" till 1845. Not hugely popular.'

'I've seen glasses nowadays that take half a bottle,' rumbled the colonel.

'Oh, we have those in the States – to facilitate breathing.'

'Facilitate boozing, more like!'

'Fleur read history at Girton,' said Reggie, filling Shandy's glass. 'Girton College, Cambridge. She was one of the first women undergraduates. Inspired Sebo.'

'A pioneer,' said Shandy, raising her glass.

'One of the few women, more's the point,' Fleur replied. 'So there was no competition for the chaps. How on earth do you think I snared dear Sebo's uncle?' Fleur gazed at her sherry. 'Francis Drake brought three thousand butts of this stuff back from his raid on Cadiz in 1587.'

'How much is a butt?' asked Reggie.

'About two cheeks,' murmured the colonel. 'Hee-hee-hee.'

'One thousand and eight pints,' said Shandy, who had whipped out a smartphone. 'A lot of these.' She raised her weeny glass again.

'Exactly. London was awash with the stuff. Elizabeth I adored it, and the Court and everyone else followed suit.' Fleur noticed the colonel adding more gin to his gin and tonic.

'And your gin, Colonel.' She tried to draw the old soldier into the conversation. 'That's a legacy of the War of the Spanish Succession.'

'Eh?'

'From our Dutch allies: hence "Dutch courage". Unfortunately it was so cheap and strong, it became a craze, like absinthe in Paris after the Algerian War.'

'Or crystal meth,' said Shandy.

'Except this was legal, and dirt cheap: "Drunk for an 'a'p'ny, dead drunk for a penny." Until they brought in a savage tax.'

'Terrible thing,' said the colonel.

'War?' said Shandy, shaking her head.

'Tax,' he said.

'And yet it's the key to our national love affair with port.'

'What?'

'Tax. And funnily enough there's a Spanish link: the War of the Spanish Succession again.'

'Ah?' The colonel was being almost agreeable for a change.

'Louis XIV had designs on the Spanish throne, which would have given him control of France and Spain, scaring the wits out of the rest of Europe. At the Treaty of Methuen in 1703, we promised to obstruct those dastardly plans in exchange for Portuguese troops, the use of the port of Lisbon, and no duty on British wool in Portugal or its colonies.'

'The Portuguese and British are hereditary allies. Every soldier knows that.'

'We agreed to slash the duty on Portuguese wine, while maintaining it on wine from France and its allies and satellites.'

'Not that onerous, I suppose, as they produced no wool and we produced no wine.'

'Precisely. The treaty lasted till 1836. And that's how we fell in love with port.'

'That and the taste.' He took a gulp of gin. 'And the fact that it ages so well. Tucked away in the cool and dark. You can give someone something quite affordable and ordinary and ten, twenty, even fifty years later . . . it's delectable.'

'Charming. I'd never thought of it like that.'

'Otto at the Spatchcock says the 1815 Ferreira is still superb. Think of that: the year of Waterloo. Not that anyone drinks port these days.'

'What about passing it to the left? Why do we do that?' I asked. 'No one seems quite sure.'

'To wrong-foot wallies like me, who can't tell their right from left,' Reggie laughed.

'To leave the sword arm free,' said the colonel.

'Quite right,' said Fleur.

Pam swooped in, whispered in her mistress's ear, and scooped up the flowers.

'Look at these colours! Aren't they wonderful?'

'Amazing how *vulgar* nature can be sometimes,' said the colonel, who thought they were from Tommy.

Sebastian sidled past and plunged the toasting fork with a candle stub on each tine into the fire, and left it there. The flames flared up momentarily as the wax caught, and then subsided.

'What was that?' asked Reggie.

'Puggle the candles in the bog a few times and the wax picks up the shot,' Sebastian explained. 'They don't teach you that at shooting school.' Reggie steered Shandy away to meet Jane, and Fleur rose from her chair and clapped her hands.

'Pam has just reminded me that I promised Brian I'd have you fed and watered by two fifteen,' she bellowed. 'So we'd better go in for lunch: muntjac and mash and Pam's incredible gravy.'

Brian had worked on the meat counter at Doubledays before he became a keeper, and no one knew more about hanging and butchering deer. The beaters had shot several muntjac before Christmas, a perk of the job, and we were having the fillets, as tornedos. The guns served the women and then themselves.

Very light on calories, venison, Reggie assured us, as he and I avoided the potato and took heaps of peas and carrots. Tommy made a hole in his Mount Vesuvius of mash and swamped it with gravy, a truly heroic helping.

'Now that's what I call an American plateful,' the colonel barked at Shandy, perhaps trying to make amends for disparaging her flowers – Pam had put him straight – and in the light of her business interest in books. She blinked. 'Wouldn't you agree?' he persisted. 'Everything's on a different scale: huge. Skyscrapers, lorries, servings of food.' He attempted an American accent. 'It's a mighty big place.'

'I guess it is,' she said.

'This gravy's unbelievable!' Sebastian chuckled. 'I really must get Pam to tell me how she does it.' The little coins of meat were exceptional too, melting on the tongue like gamey butter.

'Blood,' said the colonel. 'That's how you make good gravy: stock, wine, jam and blood, lots of it, and this is *very* good gravy.'

'I find it terribly hard to think of you three *bons viveurs* confining yourselves to greens and gruel,' trilled Fleur, patting Reggie's arm. 'Isn't there enough doom and gloom out there already? It's a horribly joyless way to behave, almost selfish. You don't need to lose weight, George and Reggie, and Sebastian looks like a film star. Always has.'

'Does indeed,' muttered the colonel. 'Oliver Hardy.'

'It's Reggie's turn to be selfish for a change, Fleur,' Jane replied. 'He spends his life thinking of others. The doctor said he has pre-diabetes.'

'Pre-diabetes? How bloody ridiculous,' guffawed Sebastian, prompted to take some more Argentinian Malbec from the very fine decanter. 'We've all got pre-something.'

'In your case a pre-black eye,' Jane snapped. 'And George isn't being selfish, he just wants to stop snoring.'

'Ignore Sebastian, darling,' soothed Reggie. Sebastian pushed the decanter her way, raising his eyebrows and joggling his eyes. 'It is weird though, Fleur,' Reggie continued, 'how so many people seem to be offended by the fact one's dieting; as though it were some kind of personal criticism or rebuke.'

'I have a different problem,' said Sebastian. 'People keep telling me how incredibly well I'm doing, when I'm not. Everyone was gushing over my progress at that last watercolour auction. I didn't have the heart to tell them I'd only lost four pounds. I'm obviously filed under "jumbo" in everyone's memory bank. They think of me as a balloon.'

'Sounds about right,' said the colonel.

'And then several really skinny people, people a fifth my size, who had already told me I wasn't fat at all, solemnly informed me that *they* needed to lose weight. Bizarre.'

'I get that a lot,' said Tommy. 'And I think I understand it. Because you're fat you're essentially inferior, and therefore exempt from the normal rules. Being slim and superior themselves, they're subject to more exacting standards.'

'Well, I *have* done well, but I've still got miles to go and yet, I agree, I've lost count of the number of people who've told me not to lose any more, or lose too much.'

'You're being oversensitive, Reggie,' I said. 'No one with any manners is going to tell someone he needs to lose weight. Especially someone who's been dieting for weeks and weeks.'

'Maybe.' He sighed. 'I must say I was appalled by that promotional video thing. That's not how I think of myself.'

'But that's you,' Fleur insisted. 'The you we love; the you *everybody* loves. How could we want less of that?'

'I want less of that. I no longer want to look like the twerp I see in the mirror.'

'Want to look good naked,' said the colonel.

'I'd settle for looking good dressed,' I said.

'I'd settle for being able to *get* dressed,' said Reggie. 'I'm simply too fat. I have to sit down to put my socks on.'

'And Reggie opened the batting for Scottish Public Schools,' said Jane, proudly.

'Can't believe that required much . . . agility,' the colonel sniffed.

'You don't need to run if you only hit sixes,' Jane snapped back.

The colonel turned away, catching Shandy's eye. 'Cricket,' he explained.

'I'm more familiar with baseball,' she told him.

He nodded. 'Of course. Fascinating the way adult Americans can't get enough of our English children's games: rounders and netball, for instance. Something to do with being such a young nation perhaps? Childish.'

'Is it true cricket was invented by the French?' Shandy replied with a slight edge to her voice, though still smiling.

'Blasphemy!' laughed Reggie, anxious that everyone remain friends. 'French cricket is a different game entirely.'

'Children's game,' said the colonel.

'I did see a game once, in California, a game of English cricket, but it never seemed to end and I'm not sure I got all the rules.'

'Incomprehensible,' said the colonel. 'Supposed to be: like medicine or the stock market, deliberate gobbledegook to keep outsiders in the dark.'

86

'That's not fair, Val,' said Tommy, who was already helping himself to seconds. He wasn't called the biggest stockbroker in London because of the size of his funds. 'Where's the gobbledegook in buy or sell? It's figuring out *what* to buy or sell that's the difficult bit.'

'And you've done very well for me, Tommy,' said Fleur. 'Thank you.'

'How *do* you do well in the stock market, Tommy?' Shandy asked deferentially.

'Depends if the client wants to eat well or sleep well,' he replied.

'No guesses what you plumped for,' said the colonel.

'Take your profits. Cut your losses,' said Tommy. 'Don't be greedy. Don't be proud.'

'And be nice to your aunts,' said the colonel, with a smirk at Sebastian.

'And what about television, Shandy?' Reggie enquired, deciding never to ask the colonel again. 'Or retail. How do *you* do well?'

'Going for it, one way or another. Make the decision and then get behind it one hundred per cent. All or nothing: A big yes . . . or a big no.'

'Leadership,' said Tommy, approvingly. 'Big responsibility.'

Mikey started retching under the table. Shandy reached for her handbag on the floor by her chair. A trumpet sounded, sweet and clear, growing louder and louder.

'The *Antiques Roadshow*,' said Fleur, looking puzzled.

'My cell phone,' said Shandy, standing up and frowning into her bag. She fished out the telephone and turned it off.

'I *am* sorry. Peter's waiting.' Before anyone could offer even token resistance, she walked round to Fleur and took her hand.

'Goodbye,' said Fleur, as the men realised what was happening and pushed back their chairs. 'Thank you for the flowers.'

'Thank you. Thank *you*. It was a pleasure meeting you all.' She turned to go and nearly collided with the diminutive colonel, who was nipping across to see if there was any venison left. She held out her hand. 'Have a nice day,' she said.

'Have a nice . . . trip,' he replied, hesitating for a second before accepting her grip.

'I will. I love England.' She squeezed his hand. 'Everything's so *little* and so *old*.' Reggie escorted her out.

'That was heaven,' said Jerry. 'Eating Pam's venison to the sound of trumpets.'

'Chatting to Shandy Madison to the sound of trumpets more like,' said Tommy. 'What a corker.'

'She is rather heavenly,' agreed Fleur. 'And a real businesswoman.'

'Neither one thing nor the other,' said the colonel.

'Reminds me of Mary Tyler Moore,' said Tommy. 'Very sweet-natured, Mary Tyler Moore – upbeat, too. I wonder what happened to Dick van Dyke?'

'Anyone want the last piece of venison?' said the colonel, sliding it onto his plate.

'Yes, please,' said Sebastian.

'Too late,' said the colonel.

*   *   *

88

There was only one drive after lunch and the women decided not to come out in the rain. It was hard to see the peg numbers in the shadow of the wood, and as the rain increased I jammed on my sou'wester. I was supposed to be on the edge of the drive, rather out of things again, but Reggie, generous host as ever, swapped his peg with mine. I left my dogs with him and plodded off into the centre.

A woodcock jinxed and jerked out of the wood, a whisk of dark against the trees, and I decided to leave it. Something puked noisily at my feet. I looked down: Tommy's dog Mikey. What the hell was he doing here? Tommy always let him potter from the gun wagon to the pegs at his own pace. He enjoyed the ramble and snuffle and at his age and in his condition could hardly disrupt the shoot. Seeing my bulk and hat as I passed he had taken me for Tommy. When two more woodcock came over, I let fly at them both.

When we were back at the yard we towelled and watered our dogs and thanked the beaters and Brian.

We could see Fleur and Jane through the hall windows, nursing a giant teapot by the fire. We trooped in by the gun-room door, dumping our guns and washing our hands. Colonel Derek's mobile rang and he scuttled back outside.

Supervised by Fleur, we helped ourselves to tea, Reggie and I keeping our distance from the carrot cake, biscuits, brownies and crumpets. The crumpets, sodden with melting butter, were in a covered silver dish kept warm by a little fat candle. At last Brian came in and accepted a cup of tea and a crumpet.

The colonel dashed back through the door.

'Did I see Brian with a crumpet?' he said eagerly.

'Too late,' said Sebastian, taking the last one and folding it into his mouth. He bent down, chewing heavily, face greasy with butter, and drew the toasting fork out of the fire, proffering it like a rapier. There was something round and blackened at the end of each prong. He swallowed hard and took a deep breath. 'But can I offer you a chestnut?'

CHAPTER 4

'A desperate disease requires a dangerous remedy.'

Guy Fawkes

I left my office at seven that evening, reached the Spatchcock a few minutes later, and found Reggie and Sebastian in the hall staring at the wall. Fat Jack, the face of the club since time immemorial, had gone. He had been replaced by a painting of a thin man in a suit and academic gown, with one hand on a globe and the other in his pocket.

'It doesn't make sense,' Sebastian murmured. 'He's mad.'

'What is it?' I asked. '*Who* is it?'

'Johnny Pinion,' said Sebastian. 'The chairman.' He turned to Reggie. '*What* did he say?'

'He said Jack gave the wrong impression, in this day and age; set the wrong tone.' Reggie sounded as bewildered as Sebastian.

'And what's the right tone?' Sebastian asked. 'A pocket-billiards-playing geography buff?'

'Of course we ignored him. The committee took it for granted ... He obviously ...' Reggie took out a handkerchief

91

and wiped his nose, '. . . didn't get the message. It never occurred to us he might be so thick skinned.'

'Thick skinned? He could win an arse-whipping competition with a rhinoceros!'

'He could. But he can't beat the committee – ' Reggie tucked away his handkerchief – 'for long.'

'Can't we impeach him or something?' Sebo demanded.

'We're not a democracy.'

'First the wine committee, then the soap.' The amber squirter bottles in the boot room had not gone down well. 'The fires.' A notice on the hall board informed members that the coal fires were to be converted to gas. 'What next? Paper plates?'

And then the chairman himself pushed through the front doors in a blast of cold air. 'Look!' bellowed Sebastian. 'There *is* the bastard! Pinion! What the hell's going on?'

The chairman recoiled momentarily and decided not to take his coat off after all. Smug and mawkish, his automatic response to Sebastian's howl of rage and popping eyes was a knowing smile. A student magazine had once written of his razor-like intellect; a razor more than capable, he believed, of trimming back this lunatic fringe. He stood his ground.

'Sebastian. Reggie,' he said breezily, composure restored. 'I can't stay. Just popped in to sign some papers.'

'What have you done with Jack?' demanded Sebastian. 'What on earth were you thinking?'

The chairman took the bull by the horns. 'Those at the helm of the club have decided it's time for a change.' He made a conscious effort to keep smiling. It was not returned. 'Nothing stands still.'

'Bollocks,' said Sebastian.

'I thought you of all people, er, Sebastian, as a dealer in fine art, as a connoisseur, would appreciate the upgrade.'

'Upgrade?'

'It's not as if Jack was a proper picture, or a real painting even, just a giant coloured print.'

'*Was* a proper picture?' Sebastian seethed, looking really angry now. 'Jack's been here for ever. He *is* the Spatchcock. What have you done with him?'

'Nonsense,' continued the chairman, as firmly as he dared. This was the absolute limit. 'He's just some chap. We have no idea who. Probably, almost certainly, nothing to do with the club at all: just some anonymous fat chap. We decided ...' The chairman took in Reggie's increasingly thunderous expression and checked himself. There were only so many maniacs he could cope with, after all. '*It* was decided that such a public space should be filled by a proper portrait of a prominent member, preferably by a good – or even great – artist.'

'So you chose ... yourself. Talking of prominent members.'

'It's a Freud. One of his largest.'

'Since when has artistic merit been based on square footage?'

The club secretary softly descended the stairs. Fighting the urge to kiss him, the chairman accepted a proffered folder and quickly signed three pages. He handed it back and rubbed his hands. 'I'm afraid I'm expected elsewhere,' he said clearly and slowly, as though humouring a drunk or madman. 'Goodnight.' He paused, failed to salvage the smile, and bolted.

'I would have throttled him,' Sebastian snarled, 'if it wasn't Lent. What the hell has he done with Jack?'

Reggie steered him to the bar and ordered a gin and tonic and two glasses of wine. 'It's a straightforward misunderstanding, Sebo. He doesn't realise what Jack means to us all. When he does it'll be sorted in a jiffy. What's clear . . .' he said, taking the gin and tonic from Henry and placing it in Sebastian's hand, '. . . is we can do nothing till tomorrow. We'll put together an action group.' This was Reggie's solution to everything, from blocked footpaths to potential eyesores. He shepherded us back away from the bar. 'So let's get weighed and go and try out George's new restaurant.' He gently barged Sebastian towards the boot-room stairs and nudged him on to the first step. He started down. Henry followed with the wine.

'*Fuck!*' Sebastian gasped when we got to the bottom. We had found Jack. He was hanging above the mirror over the sinks. 'I can't believe it! Consigned to the crapper after two centuries. The man's potty. Vindictive!'

'Incredible,' agreed Reggie.

Sebastian was literally reeling. He staggered to the sinks, put down his drink and clung on.

'It's a mistake, Sebo. This is *our* club. We'll sort it, soon, I promise. There are procedures, mechanisms, for this kind of thing, but they have to be done properly. Isn't that right, Henry?'

'Without a doubt, sir,' Henry agreed.

'The girls have come all the way down from Essex and George has got us a table at Mintons. Hang up your jacket, Sebo, and let

Henry record your weight.' Henry jerked down the lever on the scales and Reggie bundled Sebastian out of his jacket. He allowed himself to be parked on the leather bench, until Henry read off his weight.

'That's it!' he exploded, scrambling straight off again. He had lost nothing, not a single ounce in two weeks. 'I've had enough!' He snatched up his jacket and stomped back upstairs.

We made no attempt to follow, and moments later I discovered I had not done much better, having lost just one pound.

'One pound after two weeks of incessant hunger and semi-permanent rage; it beggars belief!'

'It's called "hanger": hunger anger: anger caused by hunger. I read about it in the *Mail*,' Reggie explained. 'As opposed to real anger which . . .' He looked up at Jack and ground his teeth. '. . . has more tangible causes.'

Reggie had gained eight pounds. Reggie had *gained* eight pounds!

'*What!*' Neither Henry nor I could believe it. After eight weeks we took Reggie's relentless progress for granted. 'What have you been eating?'

'It was the holiday,' he groaned, too abject to defend himself. Reggie and Jane had spent the last two weeks in Thailand.

'Sorry, Reggie. I should have asked. Was it awful?'

'It was the best! The hotel was paradise, the food superb. And, I thought, safe. Fruit juice is good for you. Everyone knows that. And the fruit itself – at least five different types of banana, and pineapples, mangos, berries. But they must have added sugar to everything, even the fish. We spent hours swimming. I was being so *good*!' He put his jacket back on. 'I gained a stone in ten days. Fourteen pounds!'

'Just eight.'

'No. I've clawed back six since we got home. I was sixteen stone seven on Saturday. Couldn't believe it! Jane was shockingly unsympathetic. And it was her who banned me from weighing myself out there. Took the batteries out of the scales.'

We trudged back upstairs. Sebastian was waiting for a pack of cigarettes at the bar. The colonel was glaring at the new portrait.

'Lambert?'

'I'm as appalled as you are, Valentine,' Reggie sighed. 'But there's no point screaming and shouting. I'll call an emergency committee meeting tomorrow.' He looked up at the painting again. 'Can that really be an Aertex tie? He's not even very well hung.'

'I assumed that was the way the trousers were painted,' said the colonel.

'I meant the actual picture not . . .' Reggie closed his eyes. 'It's wonky.' He pushed the bottom left-hand corner to straighten it.

'Let's go,' said Sebastian, unwrapping his cigarettes, and we followed him onto the street. 'Can we get a taxi?' he asked, dragging the smoke down deep. 'Once I've had this? I want to be as far away as possible when the colonel comes up from the boot room. How much did you lose?'

'A pound,' I said.

'Nothing,' said Reggie. 'Put on eight.'

'Put on eight? *Put on!?* Well that's some consolation, anyhow.' He flapped at a taxi on the other side of the road with no real hope and it swept round in a perfect U-ey for us. 'Hols not too bad then?' he asked as he stamped out his fag and opened the door.

'Too many bananas,' Reggie replied, climbing inside.

'Story of my life,' said Sebastian.

As it was so close to Valentine's Day, I had cajoled Fiona and Jane into joining us for supper. They were meeting us there.

'You can't go wrong with fish,' said Reggie hopefully as we clambered out of our taxi opposite a giant illuminated lobster. 'When you're dieting.'

'And I'm the bloody lemon as usual,' moaned Sebastian, slightly cheered by Reggie's hiccup. 'Not that I'll be able to eat anything now. Do you know – till I was thirty, I never ate a decent bit of fish that wasn't wrapped in newspaper? Except fish fingers, I suppose. And kippers.'

'A politician and someone else almost famous pushed ahead of us.'

'Well, it seems your luck's about to change,' Reggie chirped, 'if the quality of punter is anything to go by.'

'"Eat like a celebrity", eh Reggie?' Sebastian sighed.

We were shown straight to our table, where Fiona and Jane were already nursing aquamarine cocktails.

'What are those?' asked Reggie.

'Not sure,' Fiona replied. 'On the house. Moscow Mules, we think.'

'Delicious,' said Jane.

'We've just had the most awful time at the Spatchcock,' said Sebastian, impaling four olives on a cocktail stick.

'You mean Reggie's blip?' said Jane.

'No,' Sebastian said testily. 'Johnny Pinion.'

'No. Please,' said Jane. 'Not Pinion again. I want to hear about the wedding plans.'

'But—'

'*No*,' Jane insisted. 'The wedding.'

Sebastian drew the olive bowl closer.

'Mary and Natasha are sorting all the finer details. I've been pretty much sidelined. Though I have booked the College Chapel.'

'Fantastic!' said Fiona. 'It's by far the prettiest. And right on the Backs. And I gather you've found them the perfect present?'

'Short of a house or a million pounds.'

'A picture, George said.'

'That's right. You're staying at Reggie and Jane's tonight, aren't you? Come round tomorrow and have a look before I send it off to be cleaned. It is lovely.'

'A future heirloom.'

'What a happy thought.'

'Natasha will be a brilliant mother.'

'She will, won't she? She'll have such fun. I loved it when they were little,' he said sadly. 'When we were still a team.'

'What do you think, Sebo? The salmon, oysters or whitebait?' Jane said quickly, signalling to a looming waiter with long hair and a pointy beard and moustache, like a musketeer.

'The trouble with Mary and me – ' he accepted a menu from the waiter – 'is that we started with the happy ending.'

'That's why your girls are so happy.'

'Thank you, Janey.' He gave her a crooked smile. '*You* don't change.'

'Of course not,' she replied, squeezing Reggie's arm. 'Too thick.'

'Thanks, darling,' said Reggie. 'What'll you have to drink, Sebo?'

'Have I not even had a drink yet?' Sebastian laughed.

'Not here, but you will, Sebo. You will.'

'Bloody Mary.' He handed the menu back to the waiter. 'Though of course I'm not saying it was her fault.' None of us said anything. 'Better make it a double, please. Thank you, and spicy.'

When our drinks came, we ordered the food. Sebastian and I chose oysters and the girls whitebait. We were astonished to learn that Reggie had already ordered online.

'Why?' asked Sebastian. 'That takes away half the fun.'

'I ordered this morning, after breakfast when I was feeling relatively full, and reasonable – open to reason. Eating is a reflex: illogical. I mean it's instinctive, not rational. Too dangerous to wait till the evening when I'm hungry, had a drink or two and, as you say, having fun.'

'Can't let yourself have fun,' said Sebastian.

'Can't let myself slip back, Sebo, after all these weeks.'

'He was so fussed he went online for tips. Didn't you, darling? Psychological tips.'

'What did you find?' asked Sebastian.

'Order online.'

'Boring.'

'Try to get a thin waiter or waitress. You'll order less.'

'Interesting.'

'Hungry people fancy fat people.'

'Told you,' said Sebastian.

'Jane and I had an idyllic time in Thailand. The Thais are the nicest people on the planet. But I blew it, big time. I *am* getting back on track.'

'Well done, darling,' said Jane. 'I'm proud of you. It was a great holiday, though.'

The waiter returned to tell us all the oysters had gone, except the six reserved by Reggie. Reggie apologised.

'No, no, no,' said Sebastian with mock stoicism. 'That's the way it's always been: the first man gets the oyster. The second man gets the shell. You're not a portable-bog baron for nothing.' The waiter recommended the whitebait.

'You have my oysters, Sebo,' said Reggie, sweet as ever. 'I'll have the smoked salmon: more dietary.'

'You are staggeringly unselfish, Reggie,' said Sebastian. 'But as I know you get a kinky kick out of it, I feel obliged to accept.'

'Swine,' said Fiona. 'George tells me you've opted for a picnic on the river, after the wedding.'

'Yes.'

'Perfect. You know George is a master punter?'

'So's Reggie,' said Jane.

'Though rather slow,' Reggie cautioned. 'Duck flighting with Jack Emson.'

'Milo's organising the punts. I'll tell him we've got some more muscle.'

'He seems a sweet guy,' I said. 'And on the ball.'

'Hope so,' said Sebastian. 'Innocent, ardent and solvent, at any rate.'

'And nice looking,' Fiona said.

'Tall and young anyway,' Sebastian conceded.

'And clearly bright. What with Cambridge and everything.'

'Seems bright enough. Certainly kind and besotted.'

'Well, there we are then. What more could you ask?'

'Nothing,' said Sebastian, breaking into a smile. 'Absolutely nothing.'

The oysters, whitebait and salmon arrived.

'I shouldn't have oysters anyway,' I said, trying not to actually drool on Sebastian's plate.

'Why?' asked Sebastian. 'I thought one couldn't go wrong with fish?'

'I'm fed up with being hungry, so I'm switching to the Atkins tomorrow, which means cutting down on carbs instead of calories and, bizarrely, though most fish have virtually none, some shellfish, like oysters, have rather a lot. A single oyster has twelve grams of carbs – more than half the daily Atkins allowance.'

'Typical,' snorted Sebastian as he added lemon and Tabasco. 'First law of dieting: if it tastes good, forget it!'

'Not the first law of Atkins. Atkins positively encourages fat: chock-full of flavour.'

'Like what?'

'Like bacon, nuts, cream, olive oil, butter, cheese, mayonnaise.'

'Mayonnaise?'

'Of course. And as much protein as you like.'

101

'I did look into it when I was doing my research. It's not just low carb, it's high protein, isn't it?'

'You can never get enough protein. One of life's building blocks. From *protos*, first. Muscle is protein so you can go bonkers on meat. And eggs.'

'But no chips. Isn't that right, George?' asked Reggie, obviously sceptical. 'And no fruit, beer or bread. It doesn't seem right somehow, cutting out fruit and bread.'

'And isn't it meant to give you frightful breath and gale-force wind?' asked Sebastian.

'I'll find out tomorrow,' Fiona said.

'That'll put the snoring in perspective.'

'Shut up, Sebo. Masses of my friends have done the Atkins, and the best thing is you don't get hungry. That's the point.'

'The thing is your body doesn't like change,' I said.

'Of course not,' Sebastian agreed.

'And suddenly cutting out carbs in the initial two-week start-up phase, when you're trying to get your body to burn stored fat instead of the carbs you used to eat, gives the whole system a bit of a jolt, not least your gut.'

'Leading to "digestive mayhem"?'

'Possibly.'

'So what about the filthy breath then?'

'The ketones produced by ketosis . . .'

'The what?'

'Atkins calls the fat-burning stage – the state in which the body burns fat for fuel – "ketosis", and the product of this fat burning, ketones, come out in your breath and pee.'

'Ketone breath? That's a new one.'

'Not just breath. The book recommends drinking eight glasses of water a day to help piss it away.'

'Doesn't really sound my cup of tea.'

'It's only for two weeks. A couple of weeks on the start-up phase, then you go on to the induction phase, when you're allowed twenty grams of carbs a day, and then on to the ongoing phase, gradually increasing the carbs until you stop losing weight.'

'All sounds thoroughly unhealthy. Unnatural. And didn't Dr A. die of a heart attack? Weren't there some horrible pictures of him in his hospital bed, fat as a barrel and out cold?'

'Aren't most pictures of comatose invalids fairly horrible?' I bridled.

'How old was he?' said Jane.

'He was seventy-two, and yes, apparently he did have a dicky heart, but caused by a virus, not skipping fruit, and he actually died from a bang on the head. He was in a coma for ages, immobile in a hospital bed, which everyone knows makes you balloon.'

'I suppose it does,' said Sebastian, draining his glass.

'No one looks their best in a coma.'

'Except Snow White. And Sleeping Beauty. And—'

'Give the poor chap a break.'

'Whether you feel inclined to give him a break or not, the point is, for hundreds of thousands of people, his diet's worked,' said Fiona. 'And you don't cut out fruit for ever, just to start. You've got to read the book, Sebo.'

'I will. Can you lend it to me?' He dispatched his last oyster with a muffled crunch and then mopped at the empty shells with a piece of brown bread. 'Can we have another bottle of this Sauvignon, please, George?'

'Of course.' He beamed at the musketeer and held out the empty bottle.

The second bottle came with the main courses: Fiona's breaded goujons of sole, Jane's tagliatelle vongole, reeking of garlic, and Sebastian's whole cold lobster with chips and mayonnaise. I had bream. After a minute or two, Reggie insisted we tuck in rather than wait for his baked cod and spinach.

'Sure you don't want a chip, Reggie?' He dipped one in mayonnaise and wafted it towards him.

'I'll wait for my cod,' Reggie said firmly. 'Fish is delicious these days.'

'Fish certainly *was* revolting,' Sebastian said, bucked by the chips. 'Except good old-fashioned fish and chips, and my mother's Friday fish pie. Though that had pretty ropey ingredients: rock-hard boiled eggs; that weird yellow haddock. And about a hundredweight of liquefied spuds. We loved it though, despite the skin, bones and occasional eyeball, which at least slowed us down a bit.'

'The experts say the more slowly you eat, the less you eat,' Reggie said.

'Brilliant!' scoffed Sebastian. 'Where would we be without those experts?'

'No, let me finish,' Reggie insisted, rather miffed at having to wait so long for his cod. 'Three hundred Swedes given three

104

hours to eat the same food actually ate twenty per cent less than three hundred Swedes given half an hour.'

'Dear old Swedes,' said Jane.

'Why?' asked Sebastian.

'Oh, I don't know. They're just so blond and good looking and wholesome. And there's something about that accent—'

'Not the Swedes. The eating less.'

'It takes time for your stomach to realise it's full; something like twenty minutes. Taking it slowly cuts the legs out from under your greed before it runs away with you.'

'So maybe we should just eat stuff that slows us down, like Mummy's bony fish pie. And winkles. When did you last have a winkle? Probably full of carbs . . .' He twisted a leg off his lobster. '. . . and filthy, anyway, come to think of it. Or lobster claws.' He was finding it hard to get a purchase with the claw crackers. 'Or unshelled almonds and Brazil nuts. Maybe we should just stir pins into our grub? Ground glass would probably be going too far.'

'There's a book in there somewhere,' said Fiona. 'The Dangerous Diet?'

'What about the Difficult Diet? People love a challenge. Using chopsticks, extra-fine chopsticks, and little tiny salt spoons, and weeny blunt butter knives and those two-pronged mini sweetcorn forks. You could create a "range", including specially blunted pins, and sell them with the book. Rather fun to design: the All Handle No Prong Diet. Genius! I'm going to make millions! Maybe Natasha and Milo will get a house after all.'

'It *is* genius,' said Fiona. 'But I suppose cooking sort of does that anyway. Cooking properly: getting the ingredients, working out the proportions, preparing and combining them all. And checking how it tastes every now and then. Certainly slows you down, and fills you up a bit by the time it hits the table.'

'We can't tell our punters that,' said Sebastian. 'Undermines the whole thing.' He whipped out a pen and his red notebook and scribbled himself a note, then tucked them back away. 'I think I'd probably be a rather good cook, if I bothered. Something a bit pitiful about cooking for one, though.'

'What about Roger the lodger?' said Jane. 'Couldn't you cook for him?'

'Honestly, Jane, I don't think I could. Our living arrangements are very finely balanced. Don't want to upset the apple cart after all these years.'

The waiter returned for our empty plates.

'Any news of my cod?' Reggie ventured, with studied nonchalance. 'Surely it's ready by now?'

'You didn't order any, sir.'

'I ordered online: steamed cod. Same as the oysters.'

'I'll check, sir.' He barged through the kitchen doors and then back out again almost immediately. 'I am very sorry, sir. It was overlooked.' Reggie gaped, stunned, until a single tear slipped down his cheek. The musketeer reddened and wrung his hands. 'We can only apologise, sir. Please have anything you like. Now, sir, on us.' He tried to give Reggie the menu. 'I really am sorry.'

'No, thank you,' said Reggie, fishing out his handkerchief. 'I'll wait for pudding.'

In honour of Valentine's Day, the puddings were either pink or brown.

'I can understand the pink, it being girly and everything, but why chocolate?'

'Because it's a treat,' said Reggie, still looking sad. 'And sweet. A luxury.'

'It's about the heart,' said Sebastian. 'The Aztecs compared extracting the cocoa bean from the pod to the removal of the heart in human sacrifice. Their sun god, Quetzalcoatl, was banished from heaven for sharing it with mankind. That's why they called it *chocolatl* – bitter water.'

'In other words, nothing to do with Valentine's Day, Sebo,' Jane said. 'You do talk rubbish.'

'Why bitter water? It's a solid,' asked Reggie.

'It wasn't a solid until the good old English Quakers got their mitts on it and rinky dinked the production process. It was a drink. The Aztecs drank it cold, the Mayans hot, as did the Spanish, Austrians and English, until clever Mr Fry worked out how to make it solidify, in moulds, and his equally ingenious co-religionist, Mr Cadbury, came up with the first chocolate box in something like 1870.'

'I can never understand why someone as ingenious as your-self, Sebo, always does so badly in the Four Colnes quiz,' Jane said.

'Too clever by half,' said Reggie, waving at the waiter.

'I just remember things,' said Sebastian wistfully. 'Unless they're important.'

'Booze,' said Jane.

We ordered two chocolate mousses and four spoons. Sebastian asked for extra cream and a bottle of Sauternes. The bill, when it came, was astronomical but, thanks to Reggie, the main courses were on the house.

Sometime after midnight, the Spatchcock night porter found the chairman's portrait on the hall floor, with Sebastian pinned beneath it, unconscious. Within minutes he was admitted to the nearest A & E.

Mary, his ex-wife, called us from the hospital in the morning. We hurried round to find her and their two daughters perched anxiously on plastic chairs in a sort of flight-deck area, while the doctor talked to Sebastian behind a blue curtain.

'It's a heart attack,' Mary told us. 'According to the blood tests. He could have died. The doctor's with him now.' Tears like cod-liver oil drops leapt from her eyes, and Reggie handed her his handkerchief. 'He's such a bloody idiot! What was he doing? He's really ill! Thank God for that marvellous night porter.'

Suddenly the doctor swept the curtain back, revealing Sebastian, sitting cheerfully up in bed wearing a disposable smock and smiling. We hurried over.

Reggie and I dragged some more chairs across and everyone gabbled at once. Reggie had brought *The Times* and some grapes from the flat.

'Didn't they have a *Telegraph*, Reggie? You old leftie.' Reggie handed him the grapes. 'Thank you. I don't suppose you've got any fudge?'

Feeling rather in the way, Reggie and I left after ten minutes – there really wasn't room for seven. We returned at midday to find Sebastian alone.

'Can we get you anything?' asked Reggie.

'What I'd really love is some of Pam's fudge. I'm ravenous.'

'Find what you love and let it kill you,' said Reggie.

'So that's a no then?'

'What actually happened, Sebo?' I asked. 'What caused it?'

'I did,' he admitted. 'I popped into the Spatchcock on the way home for a pee and maybe one for the road, and of course was enraged all over again by poor old Jack above the sinks. I went back up to check there weren't too many people about and wheedled a double Kummel out of Henry before he handed over to Lukasz, the nice new night porter. Then I went back down to the boot room.

'I climbed up on to the sinks to lift Jack down, but of course they'd screwed him to the wall. I had my penknife on me, which has a screwdriver, but it was too small for the jumbo screws. Try as I might I couldn't even loosen the bloody things. I must have been at it for ages before I gave up. Tough going.

'By this time I was feeling terrible and frankly pissed, but I thought if I couldn't bring Jack up, the least I could do was haul Pinion down to where he belongs, with all the other shits.

'I staggered back upstairs, passing Lukasz on his way to check the bogs before he locked up. I knew I didn't have much time. I managed to unhook the painting, but once off the wall it was unbelievably heavy. That ludicrous Baroque frame must be solid hardwood beneath the gilt. Anyway, I teetered there, holding

109

him up by the skin of my teeth, for what felt like an age, and then suddenly had the most agonising ache in my arms, as if some giant were gripping both my biceps as hard as he could. Then the hold changed to a bear hug: unendurable pressure. I couldn't ... I keeled over and woke up here being bollocked by Mary.' He grinned. 'Heaven.'

'How do you feel now?'

'Rather good.'

'What did the doctor say?'

'Usual crap about giving up pleasure: fags, food and drink. But he admitted it wouldn't have happened if I hadn't done all that screwing ... unscrewing rather. Apparently my potassium or sodium levels plummeted or rocketed or something. But now everything's tickety-boo.' He expertly tossed some grapes into the air and caught them in his mouth like a performing seal.

'Impressive,' said Reggie, unimpressed.

'Dangerous thing exertion, as Aunt Fleur said, but no muscle damage or anything.' He offered us the grapes. We shook our heads. 'Come outside for a stogie then. I'm gasping.'

In his paper nightie, bizarrely open at the back, suit jacket and my overcoat, Sebastian led us into a room-sized lift and down to a bus shelter by the main entrance.

There were a surprising number braving the cold, patients and visitors, forlornly puffing away, one or two with drips on wheeled stands. Some of them had already encountered Sebastian and greeted him with grunts and grins. He lit up and inhaled luxuriously. We stood with him, watching smoke seep from a perforated steel pipe lashed to the nearest lamppost, a sort of

110

all-weather industrial ashtray, stuffed to the gunnels and smouldering.

'This is disgraceful!' Reggie exploded, stamping his feet. 'And freezing! These people are ill! And that lamppost is on fire. Isn't there somewhere decent to smoke?'

'No,' said Sebastian, catching sight of Mary and frantically grinding out his fag. 'Haven't you heard? They're trying to discourage it, starting with the weak and vulnerable, invalids and oldies. Watch out, the girls are back! Hello darlings,' he shouted. 'Look who's here.'

Mary had brought slippers, pyjamas, dressing gown and sponge bag, all brand new, and an offensively muscular and tanned old man, in ironed jeans and a tight, bright jersey.

'This is Hank,' she said, 'the cardiologist, from Switzerland; the best. Janey persuaded him to come along and tell us what's what.'

'Hey,' he said, raising a hand. 'Anything for Janey.' He smiled and tossed his grey quiff. He pointed two fingers like a pistol at Sebastian's belly. 'All right, big man?' and pulled an imaginary trigger. 'Sebo, right?' He had an Americanised German accent. He raised his fingers to his lips and mimed blowing smoke from the barrels.

'Comforting,' said Sebastian.

'Thank you for coming,' said Reggie.

We retreated inside and returned to the ward, where Hank unhooked Sebastian's notes from the end of the bed and went off in search of a doctor.

The ward contained about twelve beds, all rather high with a screen on an extendable arm, and a clutter of wires, tubes, panels and electrics to either side. Each had a side table, chair and adjustable Formica plank on an L-shaped stand which could be positioned over the bed for eating. Lunch was being doled out.

Having changed into proper pyjamas, Sebastian clambered back onto his bed and waited eagerly for his food, his head moving a few degrees as he tracked the progress of the trolley. Hank came back.

'It's simple, Sebastian,' he said loudly. 'Your heart was unable to cope with the combination of obesity, alcohol and extreme exertion.' He hung the notes back over the foot of the bed. 'But you were lucky. The blood tests show that your heart was virtually undamaged. So as long as you adjust your lifestyle as recommended, you could have many happy healthy years ahead of you.'

'What *have* they recommended?' Mary asked.

'Realistically he has to lose weight, quit smoking and reduce his drinking. Preferably two days off alcohol a week.'

'Not the five bloody two again,' sighed Sebastian, reaching for *The Times* and flicking through it. 'It doesn't work. Probably what nobbled me in the first place.'

'I believe the current UK guidelines are unnecessarily severe, but on the five days a week Sebastian is permitted alcohol he should confine himself to no more than thirty units in total.'

'I can't drink thirty bottles of wine in five days!' Sebastian threw down the newspaper. 'That's six bottles a day.'

'Firstly it is not compulsory,' Hank retorted. 'And secondly a unit is not a bottle, Sebastian. There are roughly nine units in a normal bottle of wine.'

'Says who? Napoleon?'

'Says the British Medical Council,' Hank replied. 'There are ten millilitres of pure alcohol in a UK unit.'

'Of course,' said Sebastian, eating another grape.

'To calculate the number of units, multiply the volume in millilitres by its ABV.'

'Its what?'

'Alcohol by volume,' said Hank. Sebastian caught another grape. 'Multiply the volume of drink in millilitres by its ABV as a percentage marked on the bottle. Then divide by a thousand.'

'Ah.'

'Aside from the impact on your heart,' the Swiss continued, 'alcohol affects your brain. Mood, memory, sleep.' Sebastian lobbed up another grape. Mary snatched it out of the air. 'And concentration. It slows you down.'

'Oh, I've always been like this.'

'Oh, please don't be an idiot, Daddy!' Natasha pleaded, falling to her knees by his bed. 'Tell him, Reggie, please! I need you to give me away in May ... And chat up all my friends ... And meet my baby. Please don't drink yourself to death, Daddy! Please!'

Sebastian stroked her hair. 'Don't worry, darling,' he said. 'That's the last thing I'll do.'

CHAPTER 5

'Nemo nisi per amicitiam cognoscitur.' (No one learns
except through friendship.)

Saint Augustine of Hippo, *Confessions*

Sebastian was sitting perkily up in bed when we visited him on
his second and final day in hospital, as round and pink and
unrepentant as ever, finishing lunch.

'You are still expecting me, aren't you, Reggie?' he said, dropping his spoon and pushing away the Formica eating plank. 'You
know I'm still coming?'

'What are you talking about?' Reggie replied. 'Coming to
what?' He flopped some newspapers and yet more grapes on
Sebastian's belly while I scrounged an extra chair.

'To the Cheesemongers' dinner, of course. You asked me at
Mintons. I'm out tomorrow and back to normal and it's not for
weeks. I wouldn't miss it for the world.'

'For goodness' sake, Sebo. You've just had a heart attack.'

'Sorry, Reggie. You wouldn't shove over slightly, would you?'
Sebastian said, trying to look round him. 'Just checking whether

Steve's having his pudding. Thank you.' He scrunched a bright red paper bag away behind the bits and pieces on his side table and sank back. 'Anyway it was an event. Cardiac event. And a one-off. I haven't felt this well in years.' Reggie raised his eyes to heaven. 'So you're not de-asking me?'

'Of course not. I'm allowed three guests: George, you and Shandy Madison. Jane and Fiona can't come: tennis tournament.'

'Good, Reggie. Just wanted to make certain you realised nothing's changed. I'm perfectly well.' He noticed two untouched trifles on the unattended trolley and stiffened with excitement until a care assistant came back and trundled it away.

'Will you stop ogling other people's puddings!' barked Reggie.

'"You know my methods, Watson. The observance of trifles."'

'What?!'

'Sherlock Holmes, "The Boscombe Valley Mystery".'

'So I'm Watson to your Holmes am I now?'

'Mrs Hudson more like.' Sebastian looked round furtively and leant forward. 'Any ramifications from the pictorial – er – event?' he said softly.

'None,' said Reggie, automatically lowering his own voice too. 'Never happened.' Sebastian settled back.

'I'm not sure whether that's good or bad.'

'Amazing you didn't do any damage to the thing.'

'Pity,' Sebastian said. 'When do we get Jack back?'

'The committee's working on it. And half the club's written to complain.'

'Like the smoking ban.'

116

Sebastian enjoyed his two days in hospital. He liked the attention, especially from his daughters, despite their lectures on drink, diet and cigarettes. They harangued us too. He got on well with the staff and other patients and had been touched by the number of visitors. Even the colonel dropped by, with a bottle of bourbon wrapped in a centrefold, claiming weight lost in hospital did not count. He was referred to Reggie and overruled. Not that Sebastian was losing weight.

'Being in hospital,' he said, 'is like a long-haul flight. It's cramped, full of strangers, the loo's a palaver, and smoking's a nightmare, of course, but it's a great place to catch up on films. Have you seen *Guardians of the Universe*? Terrific. And headphones: what a godsend. The food's regular, and not so frightful, comforting in a way, and one does get there in the end.'

'Where?'

'Wherever one's going: out.'

'Or not,' said Reggie, severely.

'Oh, come on, Reggie.' Reggie's frown softened. 'Would you do me a favour?'

'What?'

'I want to give something to Lukasz, the new night porter, to apologise for vandalising the premises on his watch and generally fucking up his evening.'

'Quite right. Poor chap's only had the job six weeks. Still on probation.'

'I've called Henry and we're in luck. He's an absolute fanatic about single malt whisky.'

'Are you sure?'

'What do you mean?' Sebastian asked.

'Well, I can never believe anyone really likes the stuff. Or can tell one from another. All equally vile,' said Reggie.

'That's what you say about beer and coffee. Your taste buds are stuck in the nursery,' said Sebastian.

'And it's not even especially Scottish, either,' said Reggie.

'So when they market it as Scotch . . .?'

'It was a sort of cult at Gordonstoun. Part of Scottish studies, which you were allowed to do on Wednesdays, with the occasional actual drink, if you were too thick for Greek.'

'Pretty much all of you then,' said Sebastian.

'And all that guff about water of life, *uisge-beatha*. The Romans called all spirits "water of life", *aqua vita*, because they used it in medicine. Whisky is just water, *uisge*, in Gaelic.'

'I think I sort of knew that,' I said.

'And you know how it caught on?'

'One of the few easily available ways of anaesthetising oneself against being Scottish.' Sebastian was still hurt that anyone in Scotland had wanted a referendum.

'Two things: Prohibition in the US, and that pest Shandy talked about.'

'Phyllo-what-not?'

'It killed all the vines in France, too, totally knackering brandy production.'

'So whisky filled the breach?'

'Whiskey was a big thing in Ireland, whiskey with an e, even bigger than Scotland. And the quality was pretty hit and miss – moonshine, mostly – until an Irish customs officer called Coffey perfected the whiskey "column still", enabling them to distil enough drinkable product to meet the sudden demand.'

'So where does Prohibition come in? You'd think it would knock it on the head.'

'During Prohibition between 1920 and 1932, the sale of alcohol was banned in the US except for "whiskey prescribed by a doctor and sold in a licensed pharmacy". Coincidentally, the very same time that Walgreens went from having twenty to having four hundred pharmacies.'

'Who are Walgreens?'

'American chemists. They own Boots.'

'You've taught me something, Reggie.' Sebastian respectfully dipped his head. 'I never thought I'd be taking history lessons from an Old Gordy, or whatever you call yourselves.'

'Always a pleasure to enlighten the ignorant.' Reggie smiled.

'But I'm pretty certain Lukasz did not do Scottish studies at school, so I've written down the name of a very rare Jura job that Henry says he was rather taken with. Berry Brothers have it in a special tube. I've bagged him a bottle, dictated a message, and paid for it down the telephone. Would you mind collecting it in the next day or two and dropping it round one evening?'

'Nothing could be easier. Done.'

'Thank you. I would do it myself but the girls are insisting on picking me up and driving me straight down to Fleur's.'

'That's sweet of them. Chance to catch up on your mah-jong.'

'What's this?' I picked up a photograph of a pig's face on an A4 slab of reflective glass.

'Mirror. Jerry brought it for me. It's Boris, his prize boar, ex-prize boar. And Tommy gave me these.' He passed over what appeared to be a pair of giant rubber clothes pegs. 'Part of a "bed pack", for "getting fit without getting up". You open and close them and get very strong hands, I suppose. Useful for twisting the lids off jars, if nothing else.' Reggie flexed them a couple of times and passed them back.

'May I have a grape, please?'

'Knock yourself out.' Sebastian tossed him the bag. 'Have two. Could you ask Steve if he's having his trifle? I never have trifle and it's something of a signature dish here. I love the cold custard.' Steve smiled from the other side of the ward and proffered his bowl. I fetched it. 'Thanks, Steve,' Sebastian said loudly. He reached for a disposable plastic cup on his side table. It was full of empty pistachio shells. He poured them on to the trifle and stirred them in, though was careful to separate the custard first.

'What on earth are you doing?' Reggie asked.

'The Difficult Diet. Fiona and I invented it at Mintons. The theory is it slows you down, allowing the "feeling full mechanism" to kick in before you've had time to scoff everything.'

'But that's your second bowl.'

'Yes.'

'And it was presumably you who ate all the nuts in the first place?'

'You can pick holes in anything. It's a work in progress. The trouble is I can't help subconsciously rising to the challenge. I definitely do start to feel full, but force myself to slog on to the end.'

'And that's one of Pam's fudge bags, isn't it?' Pam's fudge invariably won first prize at the Colneford show. She sold it in poppy-red bags in the village shop to raise money for the British Legion. Sebastian always had a stash in his flat. His lodger must have brought it.

Reggie looked at me and nodded. It was time. We drew in our chairs.

'Sebastian,' Reggie said solemnly, 'we want a word.' Sebastian waved his spoon in the air as though to bat away our formality and mumbled a nutshell into his palm. 'You've had a heart attack . . .'

'Event. My heart was not attacked, it just conked out for a second.'

'Heart attack, for goodness' sake, and you're carrying on just as before.'

'Rubbish! I haven't had a drink in two days – well, not until the colonel's thoughtful gesture, and no withdrawals either, so I'm not even addicted. And I'm hardly smoking at all. What more do you want?'

'I want you to listen to the doctors and take their advice. I want you to give up your suicidal over-indulgence. I want you to rein your drinking right back and start taking our diet seriously!'

'Okay.'

'Natasha is having a baby! Do you want to meet your grandchild? You've got to get a grip. I can't believe you had a second pudding. You ate it in five seconds flat. So much for The Difficult Diet.'

'It was difficult.'

'Not difficult enough. You're too fat. Your heart can't cope. Your family and friends love you. Brace up!'

'Okay!'

'What?'

'Okay!! You're absolutely right. I have been a bit . . . couldn't give a shit.' He plonked the bowl on the table with a clatter of nutshells. 'And I must admit I was a bit rattled by my weight before Christmas. I've discussed it with Steve's son Kevin.' He grabbed the empty bowl again and held it up to Steve, nodding in appreciation, rubbing his tummy and mouthing yum-yum. He plonked it back on the table. 'I admit the DD needs refining. Maybe dried peas or coffee beans instead of pistachio shells?'

'DD?'

'Difficult Diet.'

'Diet Dodger, more like. Another crackpot scheme to give you an excuse to keep stuffing your face.'

'The whole point is it makes stuffing your face more *difficult*. It just needs a bit of tweaking.' He looked up defiantly. We stared back, stony faced. 'I'm trying a number of things.'

'What do you mean?'

'New initiatives. For a start I'm ditching the Fast Diet and going on the Atkins . . . tomorrow.'

'What?'

'Kevin's in men's casuals at Humdingers, and they were threatening him with the kitchen department because he got too big and didn't bring out the best in the summer range.'

'Who's Kevin? What on earth are you talking about?'

'Look: Kevin, Steve's son, Steve over there, works in Humdingers, the giant shop, in men's casuals, the men's clothes department.'

'Ah.'

'Anyway, it turns out Fiona's right.'

'About what?'

'The Atkins. Kevin swears by it. The weight pours off *and* you don't get hungry. I'll miss toast and porridge and beer, of course, but console myself with berries, nuts, vegetables and vodka. I'm afraid I started cheating. It sort of crept up on me.'

'Really?' said Reggie. 'You surprise me.'

'I didn't think it would really count. Wasn't noting it, even, but I'd started keeping myself going with the occasional olive, nut, or sometimes even a crisp or biscuit on the fast days, which strictly speaking—'

'Crisps and biscuits! No wonder you haven't lost a bean.'

'It was so insubstantial, but it's amazing how it all adds up. And on the Atkins you *can* top up with olives, nuts – bacon, even.'

'Within reason.'

'He also has another strategy, to stiffen resolve.'

'What?'

'Looking as flabby, feminine and frig-awful as possible.'

'What are you talking about?'

'The three *f*s, he calls it. Kevin never really cared how he looked. He's got an angelic fiancée and hilarious twins, but he drew the line at downright repulsive. So when he realised he had to lose weight or lose his job, he went out of his way to

123

accentuate the negative: look as grotesque as possible. Skin-tight shirts and jerseys, painfully small trousers, hideous hair-cut . . . Surrounded by mirrors at work in a clothes department, his own reflection literally appalled him into losing thirty pounds in six weeks.'

'*Six weeks?!*'

'Exactly. And he's actually eating less, still shrinking. And his appetite's shrinking too. That's what so many of these diets are trying to induce, have you noticed? The Atkins, the Fast Diet, even Weight Watchers: appetite shrinkage.'

'Good point,' nodded Reggie, anxious not to do anything that might knock Sebastian out of the diet zone.

'I always assumed it was bullshit, but it's actually true. And do you know the best thing?'

'What?'

'On Atkins you can eat cheese, mountains of smelly cheese.'

'And as much celery as you can shake a stick at,' I added, puncturing his glee.

'Time for a fag,' he said.

'Do we have to?' Reggie sighed. 'It's so bloody cold and grim out there. I tell you what. Something's got to change. At least a fifth of the country smokes, despite the ban, so how can we call it a *National* Health Service when we're treating twenty per cent of the nation like bloody pariahs? Especially when they're ill? It beggars belief! I'm not standing for it.'

'Quite right, Reggie. Set up an action group.'

'A petition, I thought.'

'Even better.'

'Goes straight to Parliament. If we get more than 100,000 signatures they debate it in Parliament. It's the law.'

'You're such a *doer*, Reggie. Well done. And in the meanwhile I'm gagging for a gasper.'

'There's got to be a portable or prefab solution, a canopy or inflatable ... something. The fag companies should sponsor them. Anything's better than a kerbstone. It's a national disgrace.'

'All the more reason to suss out the current arrangements,' Sebastian rolled out of bed and grabbed his dressing gown. 'While you're here. Come on.'

Deeply proud of their history and traditions, the Worshipful Company of Cheesemongers is one of the oldest livery companies in London and naturally suspicious of change. White tie and tails are still mandatory at company dinners and the Cheesemongers' Hall is a byword for splendour and opulence.

Six weeks after Sebastian's heart attack, we changed for the Cheesemongers' dinner in the Spatchcock boot room. Despite the resignation of half the committee and the letters of outrage from so many members, Pinion's portrait was hanging in the hall and Fat Jack was still relegated to the loos, intensifying the gloom into which Reggie and Sebastian had sunk the minute we entered the building.

For a second time it was Sebastian's turn to triumph on the scales. He had piled on the weight after his heart attack, gaining twelve pounds in the two weeks he spent in hospital and then at his aunt's house. His daughters' horror at the extent and speed of the gain, shamelessly leaked by Jane, finally prompted him to do the Atkins properly, cutting right down on carbohydrates. He lost nine pounds over the following two weeks, and another eight in the next two. Reggie and I were slowing, but had still managed to lose three pounds each in the last fortnight, and were increasingly confident about reaching our targets by June.

Many of the Cheesemongers wear second-hand, inherited or hired tails for company dinners, but Reggie has always delighted in giving and spending, even more so since he became rich, and was measured for evening tails in Savile Row the minute he joined the livery. But once so splendid, they were now loose and shapeless, making him seem shabby and baggy, a shadow of his old self, as though his bulk and raffish vitality had been somehow connected.

My grandfather was taller and thinner than I am and, despite the months of dieting, his tailcoat was still tight across my shoulder blades, pulling my arms back and forcing my chest out like an opera singer. At least the hired stiff shirt was the right size, though the attached wing collar was tackily implausible, and Sebastian had to enlarge the cufflink holes with his penknife. Nevertheless, despite the feeling I might pop at any moment, once I was dressed I could sense myself adopting a sumptuous mill-owner swagger.

Sebastian's white shirt with a soft collar was a cop-out, but his second-hand tails fitted perfectly, and strapped into his cream silk waistcoat with matching bow tie, he looked the archetypal Victorian grandee.

We stepped on to St James's, unaware of the colonel a few yards higher up flailing at passing taxis. We secured one instantly, there being three of us, perhaps, bringing the colonel gibbering down towards us.

'Night, Valentine,' Reggie called as we clambered in, misunderstanding his expression: the final straw.

'Fat bastards!' he roared, stamping his feet and shaking his fists like Rumpelstiltskin. 'Preening shits! Queue-bargers!'

'Do you think he's quite right in the head?' Sebastian asked, yanking the door shut and dipping slightly below the window. 'Where on earth does he get his animosity from?'

'Jealous,' said Reggie.

Parts of the Cheesemongers' Hall are said to date from Saxon times, and the dining room regularly seats two hundred or more, and yet the modest entrance off Shackle Alley is normally easy to miss. After a minute or two in a taxi-jam, our driver suggested we might as well walk the final few yards. We soon found the hold-up: journalists spread across the road with cameras and microphones trained on an ex-mayor of New York, the current lord mayor of London, and Shandy.

Swathed in scarlet velvet, Shandy was wearing long white gloves and gems the size of boiled sweets: diamonds and emeralds. She saw us, hurried over, and barely had time to kiss Reggie before he ushered us inside, the stentorian beadle holding the door wide and commanding the journalists to 'stand right back there!' in a voice of brass.

'You look breathtaking!' exclaimed Sebastian. 'And what a lovely tiara.' She touched the emeralds at her throat. 'And necklace, and earrings and bracelet.'

'My working stones.' She smiled. 'Property of the English Channel: the prototypes for our Crystal Palace Collection. Named after your Great Exhibition of 1851. Couldn't pass up this opportunity for some pre-launch publicity.'

'They're beautiful!'

'That's what we do. What the channel does: promotes beauty. And yet Reggie tells me you're blocking our Dolls' House deal? You took a hatchet to our draft proposal.'

'I did, Shandy,' Sebastian admitted. 'The trust is a charity, not a business. I'm sorry to be a pompous arse, but I'm not prepared to compromise or take commercial risks. It's up to your lot to make us an offer we can't refuse, with cast-iron guarantees.'

'And provide the labour and the money and the entrée to America?'

'Of course. Why else would we do it?'

Heavy individual 'cards', the diner's name inked in flowing copperplate on the front of each tasselled booklet, awaited collection at the foot of the stairs. They detailed the wardens, the speakers, the music, the wines and the food, and the words of the graces, toasts and National Anthem. I picked up mine and unfolded the seating plan, my seat marked with a tiny red heraldic cheese.

Reggie gently herded us upstairs, where a man in red tails announced us to the wardens in a shattering roar. They shook our hands and nodded us through for drinks in the Court Morning Room.

Reggie seemed to know everyone, and was delighted to see them all, especially those 'in the trade', including a retired naval

128

commander reviving Essex cheese to 'knock Parmesan for six'; a woman working on asses'-milk bath salts, and a sheep farmer troubled by the 'recalcitrant rind' on his Cumbrian Roquefort. I noticed Bill Table pointing us out to his wife, tall and aloof in black taffeta. She turned away and he came over on his own.

'Sebastian,' he called as he pushed through the throng. 'Thank you for your advice. You were right about the pictures: misattributed. They were mortified.'

'So they should be, Bill. They're supposed to be the experts. Have you met Shandy Madison, the US telly tycoon? And our Cheesemonger host, Reggie Lambert?'

'No, I haven't. How do you do? But didn't I see you and your friends having breakfast in the Cock and Bull a few weeks ago? They've halved in size!'

'Reggie, George Courtauld here, another of Reggie's guests, and I are all on a diet together.'

'Well done,' the politician beamed. 'Wait till I tell Penelope. She's on the Select Committee, the Health and Wellbeing Committee. Right up her alley.'

'Shall I be the judge of that, William?' Baroness Table materialised at her husband's shoulder, sceptical and imperious. Her voice was deep and her tone arch, as if she knew what you were hiding and why.

'Honey. Can I introduce you to these three dieters?'

'Dieters? Just started, I presume? I need you, William. Come on.' She stalked off, and with a wince of apology he scurried after.

We took our drinks to a wall of glass shielding some of the company treasures, artefacts to do with the production, storage,

129

sale and consumption of cheese over the centuries. Reggie pointed out a black thread with wooden handles at each end. Not thread, he explained, wire. A cheese wire used to garrotte the notorious Watling Street Highwayman in the Great Stilton Ambuscade of 1817.

'You had a wire round your waist when we were changing, Sebo,' I said. 'What was that?'

'A belly ratchet,' said Sebastian, taking a deep breath as if to suck in his stomach. 'My own invention.'

'A what?'

'You gave me the idea, George, right at the start, when you said your waistband was like cheese wire. Can you remember? And your belt holes? Well this is a belt, too; an austerity belt, I suppose. The belly ratchet. It locks in progress: heavy picture wire round one's middle, with a simple ratchet slip for tightening as your waist shrinks, quarter-inch by quarter-inch. If you even think about seconds, it cuts you in half. And it's always there, like a hair shirt.'

'Even in the bath?'

'Even in the bath.'

'Sounds a tad insane,' said Shandy.

'Totally insane,' agreed Reggie. 'When are you going to stop coming up with these mad distractions and just get on with dieting?'

Before Sebastian had time to reply, the company archivist jostled his way across, looking concerned.

'Reggie! Reggie! You're fading away! Are you . . .?'

'Been dieting, Doctor, since Christmas.'

130

'Not tonight, surely?' His face sank. Reggie nodded. 'But the frosted Gloucester? The smoked Brie?'

'Hard cheese, I'm afraid, for now.' They both looked grim. 'Have you met my guests?' Reggie introduced us. 'I was just telling them about the Watling Street Highwayman.'

'Gruesome,' said Shandy. 'Garrotted for stealing cheese.'

'The cheese wasn't the point. Though it was three cartloads of the finest Stilton he was looking to drive away. It was more the firing of two pistols at point-blank range straight at the beadle's head.' The historian had a soft Irish accent.

'That's different.'

'Missed, as luck would have it, and it may have been no more than a warning, but John Lugge, our beadle in those days, wasn't waiting to find out. He dived off the cart, seeing the villain reloading, knocked him from his horse and whipped the wire round his neck. The windpipe was severed in the blink of an eye.'

'Brave.'

'Very brave indeed. He got a medal from the lord mayor, a cash reward from the high sheriffs, and two drums of Stilton a year for the rest of his life.'

'And ever since, our beadle carries the ceremonial gold wire at his belt, with ivory handles, in honour of his gallant predecessor,' Reggie added proudly.

'Who would have thought cheese had such a back-story?'

'They're all fascinating,' the archivist assured her.

'But Stilton in particular?'

'It has its own scent,' said Reggie.

'It reeks,' said Sebastian.

131

'No. Eau de Stilton: a fragrance for men and women.'

'The ultimate Valentine's present,' laughed Sebastian.

'It's the only British cheese with a trademark,' said the Irishman proudly.

'So it has to be made in Stilton?' enquired Shandy. 'In the same way it always has?'

'No, I'm afraid it is no longer made there.'

'Why not?'

'The trademark. It has to be made in Derbyshire, Leicestershire or Nottinghamshire.'

'And where is Stilton? Derbyshire, Leicestershire or Nottinghamshire?'

'In none of those counties. It used to be in Huntingdonshire, and now it's in Cambridgeshire.' Seeing Shandy's bemused expression, he explained. 'It's the county boundaries that moved, not the village.'

Bill Table scampered back over, nodded at the archivist, then pumped Reggie's hand.

'I'm so sorry, Mr Lambert. You've lost so much weight I didn't recognise you: nothing like the video. You're the portable buildings chap, aren't you? The cricket man? Such a brilliant initiative.'

'Thank you,' said Reggie.

The MP was a keen cricketer and had not only seen Reggie's promotional film but even attended a First Eleven match in his constituency. He asked well-informed questions and grew increasingly complimentary and enthusiastic.

'Perhaps you'd like to come to our fundraiser in April?' Reggie suggested eventually, blowing his nose. 'Sebastian will be there and cricketers galore. It's fancy dress and hopefully rather fun.'

'Definitely.' Bill looked quickly over his shoulder. 'If we're available. Such a good cause.' His wife came over to reclaim him, clutching at his elbow.

'William. Come and talk to the prime warden,' she purred.

'I'm just having a word with Sebastian and his friends, honey,' he simpered.

'Ah yes: the three losers.' She looked us up and down. 'The un-thin. I will never understand how anyone with half a brain lets themselves get fat in the first place. Knowing how unhealthy it is and how very unattractive?'

'That's a bit harsh, darling.'

'Not harsh, William, honest. The obese are weak, greedy or stupid. Often all three.'

'Stupid?'

'Of course. I can't remember the last time I met an intelligent fat person.'

'Perhaps the intelligent ones avoid you,' said Sebastian, grinning.

'Reggie's asked us to his fundraiser in April,' Bill said quickly.

'We're busy.'

'But this is Reggie Lambert: the portable buildings man who does all that good work with cricket pitches. You know? The one you so approved of? Reggie the Hut.'

'And this must be his cousin Jabba?' she said, her gaze playing over Sebastian's drum-tight waistcoat like a lecher's over a cleavage. He smiled back and she jerked away, screeching, 'The

133

mayor! *The mayor of New York!* Come on, William!' She careered off, dragging her husband with her.

'Doesn't pull any punches,' said Sebastian.

'Vile!' said Shandy. 'What a bitch!'

'I have that effect on some people.'

'You just couldn't behave like that in US politics.'

'The House of Lords. No pesky public to worry about. No elections.'

'I'd heard she was a character,' said Reggie, discombobulated into accepting a cheese straw, but recollecting himself before it reached his mouth.

'Let's hope they really are busy in April,' said Sebastian.

'I like him,' insisted Reggie, awkwardly holding the cheese straw as far away from himself as possible. 'Really clued up. Rather flattering. He wants to help.'

'She was venomous,' said Shandy. 'Foul out of nowhere.'

'Will you try a cheese straw, Shandy?' said Reggie, presenting it to her like a rose. 'A favourite of Alfred the Great's, according to company legend.' She cautiously relieved him of the stick and took a nibble.

'Mmm. Superb.'

'Are there any quail's eggs or olives?' Sebastian whined. 'I need protein.'

'No,' said Reggie.

'Why don't you tell Shandy about the Cheesemongers, Reggie?'

'Would you be interested?' Reggie asked eagerly.

'You kidding?'

134

'Well, the London livery companies are the old City of London guilds, a cross between unions, trade associations and friendly societies, which regulated their own trades, guaranteed their own standards and protected their own turf. They each had distinctive uniforms or "livery" in medieval times.'

'So livery companies,' nodded Shandy. 'I had a peek at the website. But why "company"? Doesn't that mean business rather than society?'

'We're involved in business and we are legal entities with charters and constitutions, but company in the sense of friends, companions: *com panis*, with bread. Those who break bread together.'

'The livery companions. All for one, and one for all.'

'The richest and most powerful are the Great Twelve, nearly all granted their royal charters in the fourteenth century, including the Skinners, Fishmongers, Goldsmiths, who still mark London gold and silver at Goldsmiths' Hall.'

'The hallmarks, I saw that.'

'And the Grocers, who used to control the spice trade.'

'The Great Twelve: it's got a ring to it,' Shandy enthused.

'The Cheesemongers are not the grandest, but we are one of the oldest – arguably Saxon, though our royal charter's only twelfth century. Our hall is second to none, rebuilt after the Napoleonic Wars from profits made supplying the Royal Navy with Essex cheese, and we still have a thriving industry to promote and support. We're constantly pushing British cheeses and related charities, but we very much regard ourselves as mongers – dealers – as well as makers, so we're more than happy to champion shops and imports if they're sold in Britain. We've just had a bit of a do here for Gorgonzola, in fact.'

'You're the good guys, I can see that. And this place is out of this world. What a turn-out. And nothing suits men better than white tie and tails. I love a stuffed shirt. Always have. Stuffed in a good way. It's a great look. Though Sebastian's cheating.'

'Hardly,' said Sebastian. 'Don't you like the waistcoat and tie combo? Jermyn Street's finest.'

'I was thinking more Sesame Street,' said Shandy, before we were blasted into silence by eight military trumpeters and invited to find our places for dinner.

We surged gently back out onto the landing, through a series of monumental wooden doors and on into the gigantic dining room, where two hundred and forty places were set for five courses. The ceiling, painted with the Myrtle nymphs teaching Aristaeus, the Greek god of cheese, the secrets of herding cattle, keeping bees and growing olives, was illuminated by two thousand candles in twelve chandeliers, shivering and quivering overhead.

The wardens, with fur-trimmed gowns, chains of office and nosegays against the plague, entered last, with their guests, and processed to the high table.

After grace we took our seats, opposing pairs in the middle of one of the four long thin tables arranged in a giant capital E, in honour of the Queen, and two hundred and forty Cheddar soufflés materialised simultaneously. I was next to Reggie, who was opposite Shandy, next to Sebastian. The archivist was on Shandy's right.

'Now this is what I call dining!' exclaimed Shandy. 'What a privilege, Reggie! Thank you.'

'I'm glad you like it, Shandy. I think Sebo just said no to a bun. At long bloody last, he's actually dieting.'

'Of course. You all are,' she said. 'How's that going to work this evening?'

'Well, I'm here for the company – the people I mean – not the food, so I'll eat virtually nothing, though I will allow myself a glass of wine or two, and that's pretty much it. After all these weeks, I've realised no one really cares or notices what anyone else is eating.'

'Unless they're cooking or paying,' said Sebastian. 'But George and I are here for the drink and the dressing-up. And we've gone carb free. So we don't have to worry about calories or even quantities as long as we stick to flesh, veg and cheese. No stickies, of course, or champagne – far too many carbs in champagne – but wine won't do any harm, not in these tiny glasses.'

'Not as tiny as your Aunt Fleur's. How is she?'

'Well. Thank you, Shandy. She sends her regards.'

'She didn't seem to quite approve of the diet.'

'She takes food far too seriously: something to do with rationing.'

'Rationing?'

'The government introduced rationing in the war. We nearly ran out of food, not only food, but petrol, too – all sorts of things. And then we were so broke and knackered they didn't lift the restrictions until 1954.'

'I had no idea.'

'It almost lobotomised British cheese making,' said the archivist with a shake of his head. 'And nearly killed it.'

'How?'

'Cheddar's at least as old as this livery company. Probably older. A pipe roll of 1170 records the purchase of 10,240 pounds of Cheddar for the king, at a farthing a pound.'

'That's over ten quid,' Sebastian worked out quickly. 'Bit extravagant.'

'It's named after the village in Somerset, near the caves of Cheddar Gorge where the cheese was matured.'

'Say cheese and I think Cheddar,' said Shandy, apparently interested.

'There's a reason for that. As with other cheeses, rennet is used to separate the curds and whey, but the curd is then "cheddared", that is, heated, kneaded with salt, cut into blocks to drain, and then stacked and turned. Then matured for up to fifteen months until it is firm and crumbly and shot through with calcium lactate crystals. Deliciously crunchy.'

'I could taste them in the soufflé.'

'So, as with Stilton, as with so many cheeses, Cheddar has its own lineage and traditions. Then along came Joseph Harding, a Victorian Somerset dairyman, the so-called father of Cheddar.'

'What did he do?'

'He revolutionised Cheddar making, simplified and standardised it, and exported his method to Scotland, America, Australia and New Zealand.'

'Was that bad?'

'Not initially, no. But it meant that when war came, with all its shortages and privations, the War Office saw the production of Cheddar as the most straightforward and formulaic. What do they call it now? Scalable? So they starved the other cheese makers.'

'I'm sorry?'

'Starved them of milk! Almost all the milk allocated to cheese went into "Government Cheddar".'

'I see what you mean.'

'We lost three and a half thousand cheese makers between 1939 and 1954. Terrible times: the Great Cull. Just a hundred left in the whole of the British Isles.'

'I had no idea.'

'Tragic,' said Sebastian. 'So you can imagine how seriously someone born in 1940, someone like my aunt, takes their grub. She thinks dieting's criminally ungrateful, definitely unhealthy and probably a sin.'

'Food is serious. *Diet* is serious. And it *is* a mental thing. It's about the person you choose to be, the life you choose to lead; it's about identity.'

'What do you mean, Shandy?' I asked, forcing myself not to wolf the soufflé. I too had sampled a cheese straw, several, and could feel the carbs stoking my greed. I was ravenous.

'I mean, I long ago realised that a life in television required me to look the part. And we *do* look better slim: men and women. I'm sorry, guys, but that's the truth. Excess body mass is not a good look for me, with my facial structure, and it's worse on camera. I lost twenty pounds and became the person I needed to be. I now do whatever it takes to stay there.'

'Ring a bell, Reggie?' said Sebastian.

'And now you're carb free, Sebastian? But I guess it's not going so well, if you don't mind my saying? You look . . . the same.'

'I've lost seventeen pounds!'

'Really?'

'Well, having gained twelve.' Sebastian realised he hadn't seen her since the shoot. 'Maybe only five pounds since we met.'

'In two months? I'm underwhelmed.'

'Not very impressive, I admit. The trouble is I haven't really got an incentive. What Reggie calls "the carrot".'

'Sorry?'

'You know, carrot and stick? A compelling reason, a really good motive. You had an empire to build, Reggie has his documentary and George his snoring. I'm quite happy as I am. Great.'

'Great is good.'

'I only managed to get a grip at all because my daughters have been hounding me about the wedding photographs.'

'Wedding photographs?'

'My daughter, the one having the baby, she's getting married in May.'

'Congratulations.' Shandy took a sip of water. 'And yet there's nothing you want to build? To leave your granddaughter?'

'Not that requires weight loss.'

'What does your wife say?'

'We're divorced. I suppose that says it all.'

'I'm sorry.'

'So am I. The trouble is, I've got hamster syndrome.'

140

'What's that?'

'An irresistible urge to pack my face. I literally like to eat till my cheeks creak: hence the belly ratchet. And I'm perfectly happy with the way I look.'

'That's because that's who you think you are.'

'Is that wrong?'

'Which is why you ain't busting that gut, but that doesn't mean you're happy with it inside.'

'That's the second time today a woman has dissed my look.' Sebastian laughed.

'I didn't mean . . .'

'Maybe it's a British thing, Shandy, but most of my friends aren't that bothered about weight.'

'Lady What's-Her-Name didn't strike me as so unbothered.'

'She's not a friend, and politicians are different.'

'People are the same the world over, Sebastian. They haven't changed since Adam and Eve. No one wants to be obese, whether others are bothered by it or not.' She pushed back her chair a little and turned to face him properly. 'I've been watching you all: so dry and unfeeling. Everything's a joke. You can't admit to caring about anything. But you must. Where I come from it's okay to show it. It's okay to care.'

'We care, but perhaps about different things, and show it in different ways. It's a cultural thing.'

'We're all the same . . . inside.'

'You should be a psychiatrist.'

'Too much angst . . . and litigation.' She turned back to her soufflé. 'Television suits me fine.'

'So what do *you* watch, Shandy?' Reggie broke in. 'What's *your* favourite television programme?'

'My favourite shows? The ones that make money.'

'It can't all be just business?'

'There's no such thing as *just* business, Reggie. You know that. My business is my life.'

'Now who's got the identity crisis?' mocked Sebastian.

'Look. I don't just front the English Channel. I created it and yes, I *live* it.'

'Hard work,' said Sebastian.

'Rewarding. More rewarding than I ever imagined. Work is only hard if it's repetitive or pointless. I supply the "vision", the drive, the *face*. I don't do pointless. The actual *work*, the *hard* work, I source out.'

'Sounds . . . good,' Sebastian said.

'It is. Who doesn't like shopping?'

'Well, me, I suppose,' the archivist admitted, half raising a hand.

'Sure you do. You've just been in the wrong stores.' She touched the gems at her throat, flashing white and green. 'I love beautiful things. And there's nothing on the English Channel that isn't beautiful.'

'Of course not,' said Reggie.

'Spielberg doesn't sell movies because he *gets* the public, he sells movies because he *is* the public: I *am* my viewers.'

'Ideal!' said Reggie, leaning back to allow his plate to be removed.

'Have you seen our reproductions?'

142

'No, I'm afraid I . . .'

'Take a look. You'll be impressed. And you, Sebastian: there could be a place for you at the English Channel. A highly lucrative place. Once we've signed the Dolls' House deal.'

'Bribery and corruption, Shandy?'

'Reggie said you discovered a Gainsborough.'

'Did you, Reggie?'

'Of course. Never stop boasting about my distinguished friends. Notorious name dropper.'

The cheese and ham pie arrived. Sebastian nudged his crust and potato to one side and watched as his glass was filled with claret. He took a slim enamelled snuffbox from his waistcoat and flipped open the lid.

'Ages ago,' he said quietly, sprinkling rust-coloured powder on to the cheese and ham.

'But his eyes are always open,' said Reggie. 'Aren't they, Sebo? You're a scholar really.'

'And I could use that eye, that scholarship.'

'That's very kind, Shandy, but, even ignoring the conflict-of-interest issue, reproductions aren't really my . . .'

'Even if they're better than the originals?'

'They can't be . . . as far as I'm concerned.'

She frowned.

'I assure you the quality of our craftsmen . . .'

'That's just it, Shandy. You're talking craft. I'm talking art. Not necessarily *pure* art, but we're coming from different angles.' He tasted a forkful of pie, flinched, then carefully sprinkled on more dust. 'A lot of what makes the objects I'm interested in so

143

fascinating is their history: when and where they were made; who for; how they've worn or aged; their uniqueness. I'm simply not interested in new. If they were copies, mass produced . . .'

'*Re*productions. Not *mass* productions!'

'Of course, Shandy. I'm sorry. But I suppose the truth is that I'm not much of a businessman. I like to turn a profit, but, as you say, it's the whole life I love: the collectors and the auction houses and the archives. I *do* like my life, my identity, as a sort of amateur academic.'

Shandy looked down at her plate. 'What a waste,' she said.

'I'm working on it,' he said, patting his stomach and fishing out the snuffbox again.

'What's in the box, Sebo?' I asked. 'Surely not snuff?'

'The dried and ground pods of a member of the capsicum family,' he said, sprinkling yet more powder on his food. 'Street name, chilli. I had to can the nutshells, too damn difficult, and not nice for one's fellow diners. Chilli works just as well.'

'Not the bloody Difficult Diet again,' huffed Reggie. He turned to me. 'How's Ludo, George? Talking of work. The poor benighted graduate? Got over the diesel incident?'

'I'm afraid he's been . . . "let go".'

'Oh dear.'

'He was supposed to be spending a week on the dealing desk. On the very first morning Tony, the head dealer, gave him a fifty-pound note and asked him to pop out to Marks and Sparks and get him a bacon butty and something for himself.'

'And?'

'He came back half an hour later with Tony's sandwich and . . . a penny change. Tony went ape-shit, of course.

'"What the fuck's this?" he said, holding up the penny. "I gave you fifty quid!"

'"You told me to get something for myself," Ludo pleaded.

'"So what did you get?" raged Tony, seriously pissed off.

'"A sweater," he said.'

'Poor wally,' said Sebastian.

'My client's not over the moon,' I said. 'Rather lost faith in my judgement, in fact. And the boy's father—'

'Self-sabotage,' said Shandy. 'He torpedoed himself. He's not an idiot, right? Far from it, you said. He's been pressing self-destruct. Did he want a job in finance?'

'He's got a first from Imperial and his father—'

'His *father*? Exactly.'

'I told you you should be a psychiatrist,' Sebastian tutted. 'You're a grad-whisperer.'

'Ask him to contact me at Claridge's, George. I don't believe he's the innocent you think he is.' Shandy sniffed. 'And if he isn't, I could really use some local help right now, as I was just telling Sebastian.'

'Wonderful, Shandy.' I was grateful. 'Thank you.'

'And talking of dolts, Sebo,' said Reggie. 'How's Operation Grotesque going?'

'You saw the results this evening. Eight pounds!'

'What is Operation Grotesque?' asked Shandy.

'It's all about *not* looking the part,' said Sebastian. 'Supercharging your vanity by constant reminders of how bad you look. Pitch one vice against the other, greed against pride, and shame yourself off the nosh.'

'And just how are you doing that?'

'Photographs and mirrors mostly. I have a reflective pig's portrait at head-height on my fridge door, with FREEZE PIGGY spelt out in magnetic letters underneath. I see my face gradually melding with the pig's as I approach. Stops me dead.'

'I guess it would.'

'I wear a bowler hat when I go out, which really sets off the cheeks, and "figure-hugging" shirts and trousers to emphasise the moobs and paunch. Horrible, I assure you.'

'You had me on "Freeze Piggy".'

'Though the tourists seem to like it.'

'Sure they do. An English archetype.'

'Yes. The village idiot. And I eat in front of a mirror when I'm alone so I'm subjected to every bite and mouthful in galling close-up. It's seriously off-putting.'

'Anything else?'

'My daughters have plastered enlarged holiday snaps all over my flat: me in swimming trunks, mostly, looking like a beached elephant seal; a beached elephant seal with slapped-cheek syndrome.'

'Who needs family?'

'They mean well.' They both reached for their wine glasses. 'What about you, Shandy? Do you have children?'

'I have a son: professor of Math at MIT.'

'Professor? Wow! Child prodigy.'

'Not any longer. He's almost thirty.'

'Thirty?'

'I was a very young mother, you understand?'

'Of course.'

The pudding arrived: caramelised quince and ice cream. Reggie and I refused, and so did Sebastian.

'Mmmm!' Shandy groaned, trying the ice cream. 'This is amazing. What is it?'

'All ice cream is amazing,' said Sebastian, with real lust in his eyes. 'Hyper-palatable.'

'What is hyper-palatable?' Reggie asked. 'I've heard the phrase.'

'Two parts carb to one part fat. Like breast milk.'

'I see.'

'In other words . . . irresistible.'

'What do you mean?'

'Omnivorous mammals simply won't stop eating hyper-palatable food, until it's gone, or they die.'

'I know where they're coming from,' said Shandy. 'What is this flavour?'

'Parmesan: the Duke of Wellington's favourite,' said the company archivist.

'Parmesan? You mean the cheese? Bizarre.'

'Not bizarre, Agnes Marshall: the queen of British ice cream. Cornets were her idea, made from baked almonds. She patented mechanical makers, came up with recipes, like this one, even suggested the use of liquid nitrogen. And, of course, wrote two great books.'

'I have to disagree with you there, Doctor,' said Reggie. 'Surely Maggie is the queen of British ice cream?'

'The prime minister? In what way?'

'She invented soft ice cream, according to Charles Moore, during her time as a chemist at Lyons. You know? The 99.'

'Hardly a giant leap forward, scientific or culinary.' The historian drew back in surprise. 'No taste, and a little bit sad. The soft ice cream, I mean.'

'I loved it,' Reggie insisted, but the doctor was having none of it.

'What did Michael Foot say when it came out? Typical Thatcher: "adding hot air, lowering quality and raising profits".'

'And yet there they all were, at that Labour conference in Blackpool, swaggering up and down the Promenade, sucking on their 99s.'

'They came to sneer and stayed to scoff,' said Sebastian.

'Awful chip those eighties socialists had,' said Reggie, looking longingly at Shandy's plate.

'With bloody good reason,' said Sebastian.

The 'Entry of the Cheese' was announced by another blast of trumpets. Allegedly Norman, the ritual involved standing back-to-back in case of assassins, bowing, and the exchange of knives, spoons, spatulas and cheeses. Twenty-one different cheeses were passed up and down, accompanied by a medieval stench and countless varieties of bread and biscuit.

'*Nusquam minus quam locus temperatus*,' murmured one hundred and twenty liverymen eventually.

'Never less than room temperature,' Reggie translated as he sat back down. 'The cheese,' he added, before explaining the evolution of the ancient rite and its importance.

148

'Fascinating,' said Shandy. 'You should front one of our tours.'

'What tours?'

'We're considering a joint venture with an English travel agency,' Shandy explained. 'Offering top-of-the-range tours of England.'

'Sounds fun.'

'It will be. Just as Sebastian has his list of essential books, we're compiling a list of essential places. Not just in London but Bath, Durham, Oxford, Stratford upon Avon, et cetera.'

'Wonderful idea!' Reggie exclaimed. 'A cheese tour! I could find you a few takers . . . and guides for that matter.' The doctor nodded enthusiastically.

'And other themes,' agreed Sebastian. 'What about Castles and Cathedrals? Or even Colleges? My grandmother took me to Handel's *Messiah* when I was eight, in King's Chapel.'

'Where?'

'In Cambridge. The Chapel of King's College. It blew my socks off: the space, the sound, the sanctity. I still dream of it sometimes. I'd love to do that for my grandchild.'

'I'd love to do that for my viewers!' said Shandy. 'Help me.'

One after another, Sebastian refused another pudding, a Welsh rarebit, a glass of port and a crème de menthe.

'What *is* this?' Shandy asked, pointing at the stippled soggy mat in front of her.

'Welsh rabbit,' said Sebastian, dousing it in Worcestershire sauce for her. 'A sort of Welsh pizza.'

'Savoury pudding,' Reggie added, seeing her none the wiser.

'You know what Orson Welles said about savoury pudding?'
She pushed it away.

'No,' said Sebastian.

'He said "Life's too short for savoury pudding . . ."' She tasted
her crème de menthe. '". . . and platonic love affairs."'

'Good chap, Orson Welles,' said Sebastian, filling her glass.
'Very good chap.'

CHAPTER 6

'There in no such thing as a crisis, only the next ball.'

W. G. Grace

'Stolen waters are sweet, and bread eaten in secret is very pleasant.'

Proverbs 9:17, *The King James Bible*

'Let's find out what everyone is doing, and then stop everyone from doing it.'

Sir Alan Herbert MP

To the profound shock of us all, Reggie had 'let himself down' at a stag party. Jane had inadvertently opened a message containing footage of the whole thing and she was furious. Sebastian and I initially refused to believe it, but the evidence was undeniable. We were horrified: two strippers jigged and gyrated round a room, robotically removing their clothes, occasionally stroking the head or tweaking the ties of nine avid spectators, while in the background a tenth man, apparently oblivious, methodically worked his way through fried bread, bacon, baked beans, eggs, sausages, champagne and even chips. Later he could be seen pillaging the pastry trolley. It was Reggie.

Remarkably unabashed, he refused to apologise. He had always been uneasy about strippers, he said, especially once he had a wife and daughters of his own, but had to go to support his old mate. Once there he kept himself occupied with the room-service menu. And still he lost weight. At our next weigh-in, less than a week after the stag party, two weeks after the Cheesemongers' dinner, he was down two more pounds. Sebastian claimed this as proof that the occasional blow-out 'resets the metabolism' and 'fires up the fat burners' again.

And Sebastian himself was firmly in the carb-free zone now, delighted to be following the British Dr Harvey rather than the American Dr Atkins: Dr William Harvey of Soho Square, whose prescription for his sixty-six-year-old patient, Will Banting, a coffin maker whose obesity had rendered him deaf, was set out in his 'Letter on Corpulence' of 1863.

'It's incredibly relaxed,' Sebastian crowed. '"Banting", they call it, after the poor chap whose eardrums were muffled by fat. Can you believe it? Dr Harvey allowed him "the meat of any pudding", as much "flesh" as he could manage, all vegetables except potatoes, and limitless wine, whisky or gin in the hours of daylight. It might have been made for me.'

'I told you it was worth doing your research,' said Reggie. 'Is that really it?'

'No beer or champagne, sadly. No more than one ounce of toast a day and no more than three glasses of good claret, sherry or madeira at dinner. I think I can manage that: just tank up at lunchtime.'

And it seemed that he could. At our next weigh-in, a fortnight later, he was down a whole stone since we started. I had lost double that, the prospect of sleeping on my own having made me deadly serious from the start, and Reggie was not far behind. It felt surprisingly good to be able to do up my trousers again, and ditch the tank top, but deadly serious was becoming deadly dull, now I had stopped snoring, and I was flagging. Reggie was unsympathetic.

'Of course it's boring, but that's not the point. You're thinner,' he said, looking at his own reflection in the full-length mirror beside the boot-room sinks, fists on hips like Henry VIII. 'And so am I.'

'But the diet has leached all the joy out of eating,' I whined. 'I'm quite literally boring my own arse off.'

'Don't give up now, George, just when I'm getting the hang of it,' said Sebastian. 'Banting's not boring. Gives me a kick thinking what you two are going through, for a start. Why not give it a try?'

'There's certainly nothing boring about that frightful haircut,' Reggie said. Having had his bowler hat stolen, Sebastian had resorted to a vicious buzz-cut to emphasise the full rotundity of his cheeks; cheeks that, Will Banting-like, forced his earlobes out like the chubby fins of some tiny aquatic mammal, and still met under his chin.

'All part of Operation Grotesque,' Sebastian explained. 'Invaluable when you find yourself stalking your own fridge.'

'Yes. Fleur and Pam were whingeing about that. And Roger. Why do you keep raiding the fridge?'

'Because that's where the food is, Einstein. But I've stopped that now I'm Banting: I just tuck into cheese, unshelled almonds or Brazil nuts, olives and, if seriously desperate, tinned sardines.'

'Grim. Rather you than me.'

'But you say you're bored. What are you eating? Surely you could spice it up a bit?'

'I have coffee for breakfast,' I told him, 'and broccoli for lunch every day, with a tin of tuna, or a chop, or a chicken breast, then three boiled eggs with butter for supper.'

'And nothing else?'

'Nothing else, and nothing to drink but vodka and sugarless tonic. That's if I'm not going out. If I am, I have wine.'

'I've gone turbo-boring,' said Reggie. 'I've still got to shift a stone and a half to reach my target. In ten weeks, max! At home I have porridge and a bit of diet milk for breakfast, an apple, a carrot and a banana for lunch, and a carton of soup, a tangerine and one slice of dry toast for supper. Whether I'm alone or not.'

'Whoever has wet toast?'

'Dry – as in, without butter.'

'That *is* nothing. No wonder you're losing weight. And no wonder you're bored rigid.'

'And I've given up booze.'

'What! But you've got the Cricket Ball tonight. You can't not drink at your own party!'

'Of course I can. I don't need alcohol to face my friends.'

'I always said you were a fanatic. Have you been sneaking off to AA?'

'Of course not. It's only ten weeks; earlier if I hit my target. I haven't had a drink since the stag party. I love booze, but it's a treat. And like all treats, I can do without it for a while.'

'It's not *a* treat, Reggie, it's *the* treat.'

'You *are* an alcoholic.'

'The trouble with not drinking is it takes up all your time.'

'What?'

'I did go to AA once. To please Mary.'

'What was it like?'

'You know it was founded in America, by devout Christians? But being idle but old-fashioned C of E, I didn't give that a second thought.'

'And?'

'Well, our sort of Christianity, the cosy Church of England sort of Christianity, believes in beating sin.'

'Redemption.'

'Moral recovery. Salvation! But there's another strain, a harder, American kind, Puritan, which thinks you're either damned or you're not.'

'What does that mean?'

'It means that AA thinks drunks are incurable: not in sin but in*sane*. And the trigger for that madness is alcohol. They can't be exposed to it, can't be anywhere near it, ever again.'

'If that's what it takes.'

'I disagree. Like you, I love booze. I associate it with happiness and fun, good times. I'm prepared to cut it right back, even do without for a day or two, even weeks, but I'm not giving it up altogether.'

'Each to his own, Sebo. Didn't we agree that at the beginning? Like George, I'm not finding it a barrel of laughs. I want it finished. But cutting out booze for a while is my way of getting a grip. You've got Banting, your Difficult Diet and Operation Grotesque.'

'Mmm. The first two are working, but the truth is I find it quite hard to see myself as grotesque, even with this haircut. Just not vain enough.'

'Or just too bloody vain! Are you still wearing your wretched belly ratchet?'

'No. It backfired when I blew out like a balloon on Natasha's onion soup. Which wasn't entirely Banting-friendly anyway, frankly. Not at all sure she hadn't used potato. I panicked and gummed through the wire with a pair of blunt nail scissors in her bathroom. I was being bisected. Dread to think what her other guests thought I was doing. And it turns out medium instead of extra-large boxers do the trick just as well.'

'What about your massive arse? Must chafe like buggery.'

'I've ripped up the sides.'

'Raunchy,' said Reggie. 'We'll make a Chippendale of you yet.'

The Cricket Ball, Reggie's fancy-dress party in aid of First Eleven, for which we all dress up as British heroes and heroines, takes place as near as possible to St George's Day every year, at a West End auction house. In accordance with the patriotic date and theme, the main course is Indian and a monumental carbfest, but as St George's Day also marks the official start of the

156

English asparagus season, we have asparagus between the poppadums and the curry. The chief auctioneer normally conducts the bidding, but he had a frog in his throat, and Sebastian had been nominated to step into the breach, despite his hideous haircut.

Fiona had found an empire-line dress on the sale rail in Freeport Braintree, and was going as Jane Austen, and she had hired me an electric blue velvet suit and a shirt with lace ruff and cuffs from the theatrical outfitters in Colchester. We had booked ourselves into a hotel off St James's within walking distance of my office, the party and Bond Street.

A few hours after the Spatchcock weigh-in, Fiona and I met at Fenwick's café to discuss tactics in the face of pilau rice, naan bread, onion bhajis and beer. I planned to stick to the chicken tikka, leave the rice, naan and bhajis, and drink wine instead of beer. I forced down a massive Atkins-friendly bacon omelette at the café to stave off actual hunger and then lugged Fiona's shopping back to the hotel.

As I was plugging my mobile into the charger, the ringtone sounded. It was Ludo's father, Angus. I hesitated. We had been friends since birth, our fathers both working in textiles locally. His family owned an antiquated tweed mill in Scotland, and in due course Angus had taken over the business, devoting all his energy and attention to keeping it solvent enough to sustain thirty local jobs. It was because he and his wife wanted a less draining and desperate life for Ludo that they had asked me to help find work for him in London. They had taken the disaster on the dealing desk pretty hard. What now?

'Angus,' I said, cautiously. 'Any news?'

'*Great* news, George. Ludo's found his vocation.'

'In two weeks?'

'Yes! Ms Madison. He worships her. Loves every minute. She's given him stacks of responsibility and, unless he's got completely the wrong end of the stick, he's doing rather well. She just doubled his pay.'

'Wow. Well done Ludo.'

'Jammy bastard. Anyway, I called to thank you.'

'Thrilled to be able to help.'

'I was able to help a friend too recently: a client. Got an order down to Savile Row for him at nail-bitingly short notice. Drove it down myself in the end, on Easter Monday. They didn't use all the cloth and offered to cut one of their glorious suits out of the remnant for me. I've told them what you've done for Ludo, *twice*, and they're awaiting your call.'

'What do you mean?'

'To book an appointment. So they can measure you up. I've seen you salivating at the shop windows as you walk through Savile Row on your way to your office. Fiona tells me you have a shiny new body. Now you can have a shiny new suit to go with it. Well, not that shiny. More like industrial under-felt really. I'm pinging you their number now. Ask for Dave.'

'How incredibly kind, Angus. Are you sure? That's insanely generous.'

'What would I do with a Savile Row suit? And I've got more tweed than Miss Marple anyway.'

'I'm speechless, Angus. I needed a new carrot.'

'What do you mean?'

'I mean thank you. Thank you very much.'

The hotel had reserved a tiny table for two for Fiona and me at their packed cocktail bar, where our flamboyant get-up attracted a certain amount of good-natured attention. Fiona looked like a sophisticated and sexy Emma and I, revelling in my lace and velvet, like one of the hopeless favourites on *Strictly Come Dancing*. I hoovered up the olives and macadamia nuts while Fiona tackled the crisps. After a bloody Mary and a vodka and sugar-free tonic, we set off to the party on foot.

It was barely five minutes' walk and we found Sebastian waiting outside in his auctioneer's black tie with Fleur on his arm, inexplicably dressed as Cleopatra underneath a glossy mink coat.

'You look sensational, Fleur!' Fiona enthused, kissing her on both cheeks. 'Cleopatra being a famously heroic ... Queen of Egypt.'

'Don't you start, Fiona,' Fleur snapped. 'Not Cleopatra, Elizabeth Taylor.'

'Who are you supposed to be anyway, George?' demanded Sebastian, rising to the defence of his aunt. 'Danny La Rue?'

'Not nearly thin enough yet, Sebo!' Fiona said, kissing him. 'He's Austin Powers, of course.'

'At least he's got the teeth right. And I can hardly complain, with Nefertiti standing here, bold as brass.'

'Look, you're just being unfair. Only a man would dream up this dress code. All British heroines are either dowds or frumps.

No one's coming as Elizabeth Fry or Florence Nightingale. What's the fun in that?'

'Let's get inside and see. What are we waiting for?'

'My other half for the evening,' Fleur said coyly. 'Valentine Derek.'

'I thought you were here with Sebo?'

'Certainly not. He's my nephew, for goodness' sake, and the auctioneer. He's going to spend the whole evening jumping up and down anyway. And banging his gavel or whatever it's called. Oh, look! Here is Valentine ... dressed as ... I'm not sure? Cooee! Valentine!'

The colonel was wearing a false moustache, his old green army uniform including a beret, and a duffel coat. He marched over, keeping one hand in a coat pocket. Fleur kissed him and his moustache fell off.

'Who are you, Valentine, and what's that in your pocket?' asked Sebastian, grunting as he plucked the moustache off the pavement. 'Or are you just pleased to see me?' He handed back the shred of fuzz.

'Something for George.'

'Not a CV? ... I've got it: you're Frank Spencer.'

'Calm down and stop showing off, Sebastian,' said Fleur. The colonel dabbed his moustache back on.

'No need to ask who you are, Fleur: spitting image of Elizabeth Taylor,' he said.

'And you're obviously Monty,' Fleur exclaimed, having a brainwave. 'I can see it now. Perfect.' She caught his moustache as it fell off again and put it in her handbag.

160

A taxi drew up on the other side of the road, and the colonel straightened his back with a jerk as he recognised the Spatchcock chairman.

'It's that bastard Pinion in tights. Who the hell does he think he is?'

He was dressed in Lincoln green and carrying a long bow, looking more like Mr Bean than ever.

'Robin Hood, of course,' said Fiona.

'I always knew he was a socialist,' snarled the colonel. 'I hope for his sake he's not on our table.' Reggie always hosts a table of twenty-four directly under the podium, and we were all his guests.

'Taking a table of his own,' said Sebastian.

'Bastard,' hissed the colonel, staring madly, possibly at me. I pursed my lips apologetically. He sidled up, looking fiercer than ever, and removed a thick sheaf of paper from his pocket.

'As promised,' he said gruffly, pressing the pages into my abdomen. 'Manuscript.'

'Thank you, Valentine. But I can't publish it. I'm not up to it. You deserve a proper publishing firm that can do it real justice.' The colonel favoured me with the faintest of smiles.

'We'll see,' he said. 'Read it.'

'My pockets aren't big enough. Can I collect it from you at the end of the evening?' He grunted in exasperation and jammed the paper back in his coat.

Tommy arrived dressed as Biggles, in leather flying hat and jacket, with Mikey the dog in two pairs of cardboard wings as his Sopwith Camel.

161

'Tweedledum and Tweedledee,' said the colonel.

'Are you sure dogs are allowed? They're allergic to curry or something, aren't they?' Fleur said without conviction. 'Might he not get trampled on or . . . have an accident?'

'He's just here for the beginning. I couldn't resist it. He loves parties and he hasn't got that many left.'

'Ah.'

'Ten out of ten for effort, Sebo,' he said sarcastically. 'Who are you supposed to be? James Bond?'

'James Bond?' The colonel growled. 'Trust Grace Brown to come as a fictional old Etonian.'

'Stop picking on everyone, Valentine, and come inside,' Fleur scolded. She tucked her arm through his and pulled him away.

'Why don't we go in too, Sebo?' Fiona asked. 'I'm freezing.'

'I promised Reggie I'd wait for Shandy Madison. She doesn't know anyone and he feels rather responsible.'

'How kind, Sebo,' Fiona said. 'We'll see you inside then.'

We followed Fleur and Valentine up the stairs, with Tommy and Mikey puffing alongside, and pushed through the throng in the lobby straight on into the sale room.

In a ginger beard and velvet jacket peppered with fake jewels, with slashed sleeves, puffy britches and a feathered hat, Reggie was holding court beside his table. Those who had not seen him for a while were congratulating him on his remarkable weight loss. And back in his element, surrounded by friends, joking and laughing, I realised how very much thinner he really was, and how well he looked. Not just his clothes, but his skin fitted him again, and he radiated bounce and

162

confidence. He roared approval at all our costumes, especially Mikey's, and Jane, equally regal and jewel-encrusted, rushed across to drag us over. She and Reggie were obviously friends again.

'I heard about the breakfast,' Fleur said briskly. 'Of course it was naughty but it's hardly crystal meth, is it?' Jane gave her a look that would have felled a lesser man.

'Who are they supposed to be?' the colonel demanded. 'Torvill and Dean?'

'Henry the Eighth and Anne Boleyn, of course,' Fleur shushed.

We tucked into drinks and nibbles, and were joined by Jeremy and his wife Helen as Charles II and Nell Gwyn, Sebastian, and Shandy as a willowy Lara Croft. Bill and Penelope Table arrived dressed as Nelson and Elizabeth I. I was surprised to see them at all, after the Cheesemongers' dinner, but she had repeatedly been referred to as the 'top Table' on a popular current affairs programme a few weeks previously, he being dismissed as the 'side Table'. Their attendance was rumoured to be some kind of penance on her part.

Eventually Reggie mounted the podium and brought a gavel down in a series of sharp raps.

'Dear friends, and friends of friends,' he said, and had to pause as he was cheered to the rafters. 'None of you can have been more mortified than me to discover that the generous and talented Esme is unable to take us through the auction tonight. Especially as once again we have him to thank for the use of this splendid building. Get well soon, Esme,' he bellowed, to renewed applause. 'Thank goodness for the intrepid Sebo, art aficionado, gourmand and gavel-meister, who has bravely agreed to step into his shoes this evening. Be gentle with him.

'You will find details of the lots, almost all of them kindly donated by people in this room, in the booklets on each table. You know who you are, donors. Thank you very much!

'After all these years surely everyone here understands the good their dosh will be doing. So please don't humiliate the donors by making them bid for their own lots.

'I now ask you to take your seats and prepare for the poppadums. The bidding starts with the pudding.'

Reggie stepped back down to the table. On learning from Lawrence of Arabia that his wife had been detained at work and would not be making it after all, he heaved Mikey up into the spare chair between Sebastian and Tommy.

The poppadums arrived with bowls of chopped cucumber, onion, chutney and bright pink yoghurt, and bottles of India Pale Ale, lager, water and white wine. Reggie poured himself a glass of fizzy water and Jane noticed me watching her watching him.

'He's still in the dog house,' she said, smiling. 'How on earth do you think I got him into that beard?'

'You're wonderful, darling,' he said, pulling off the beard. 'But even you couldn't make me wear the codpiece.'

'You said they didn't have one big enough.'

'You look fantastic, Reggie,' said Tommy. 'You've done unbelievably well.'

'But it hasn't been entirely plain sailing, has it, Reggie?' Fleur cautioned.

164

'I should think not,' snorted Tommy. 'If it was that easy, we'd all have six packs.' He was amazed by Reggie's success, and hugely impressed.

'Fleur is referring to a mild recent hiccup. I cracked badly, not for the first time, and got caught on camera.'

'What do you mean not for the first time?' Jane gasped.

'Where do you think that cold roast partridge and Annie's loaf went after the Cheesemongers'?'

'What? And the rest of the mayonnaise? But that was only the week before.'

'I know. But there weren't any cameras about.'

'And Mrs Cansell's birthday Baileys?' Reggie nodded. 'I *knew* I'd put it in the fridge! I looked for it everywhere. Why?'

'Just snapped. Booze, I think. Got distracted by all that cheese and had a little bit more wine than I meant to. And the morning of the stag party I'd reached a milestone. Not quite on target but a serious milestone: fifteen stone six. Two stone down! I suddenly felt I deserved a blow-out, after I'd had a drink or two.'

'The stag party *and* the night of the Cheesemongers'?' Jane said. 'I don't understand how you've lost any weight at all.'

'But I have, haven't I? And it was worth every moment.'

'But a whole loaf . . .'

'It was asking for it: so crusty and warm and moist and just sitting there.'

'Oh, Reggie.'

'I lifted it out of the bag,' Reggie reminisced. 'About the size of a moderate pith helmet, but with a real heft to it, and snorted in that irresistible biscuit-y musk. Ugh! Punctured the crust with my thumbs and prised it open, cracked it right open with a great blast of sweet, soggy pungency! Steaming and stodgy.'

'Carby!' moaned Sebastian.

'Reggie,' Jane sighed.

'I smothered one half in butter and slopped mayonnaise on the other, gouged the partridge breasts off with my bare hands and squelched them into the centre. Then, *wham!*, squished it flat and ate it in huge juicy mouthfuls, washed down with great gulps of cold Baileys. Mmmmm!'

'I'll have what he's having,' said Helen.

'Unbelievable,' said Jane. 'And you drank a whole bottle of Baileys.'

'Yes.'

'Thank goodness you've given up booze, Reggie.'

'For now,' Reggie reminded her.

'Get that in writing,' said Sebastian. 'Can't have you permanently off the sauce, Reggie. You know I hate to drink alone.'

'You could give up too, Sebo? Perhaps starting with lunchtimes? Baby steps.'

'Can't do that, Jane. Might not fall asleep at my desk.'

'Soft drinks are fantastic these days. What about that sugar-free Fiery Ginger Beer?'

'Bad news, Jane, artificial sweeteners. Shouldn't touch them with a bargepole. I have angostura bitters and soda water, if I'm going soft. I must've got through four or five crates.'

'Isn't there alcohol in angostura bitters?' she asked.

'No,' said Sebastian.

'About forty-four per cent,' said Tommy, accepting twelve spears of asparagus and hollandaise to match. 'What's wrong with artificial sweeteners, anyway?'

'For a start they're looking into this idea that they give you dementia.'

'No more than booze,' said Fiona.

'Dementia? Since when?'

'New research. Secondly, because they're sweet, your body thinks it's having sugar anyway and tells itself to store fat. So they're actually counterproductive. They make you fat! And of course you heard about the rats?'

'No,' said Tommy.

'What happened to the rats?' asked Jerry.

'Their water was laced with artificial sweetener. They had nothing else to drink, so of course they lapped it up.'

'And they gained weight?'

'Oh no, they lost weight. They certainly lost weight, because they gnawed their own balls off.'

'I've never heard such rubbish in my life,' Penelope Table exclaimed suddenly. 'Talking of balls!'

'I don't really like sweet drinks anyway, diet or otherwise,' Reggie said, sipping from his glass. 'I'm perfectly happy with fizzy water.'

'But you've heard the latest on fizzy water?' asked Sebastian.

'Let me guess,' said Penelope. 'It caused mice to talk out of their arses?'

'It made them twenty per cent hungrier.'

'Hungrier than what? Rats who'd just eaten their own balls? Don't listen to a word he says, everyone. Stop your ears.'

'Quite right, Penelope. We *can't* listen to a word anyone says about what we eat and drink because it's all wrong. The official advice we're given is simply untrue.' Sebastian leant forward in passionate earnest. 'I mean total nonsense. I've been researching diets for months now and all these reports – super-foods, medical breakthroughs – have virtually no scientific basis at all. They contradict each other.'

'Oh, come on.'

'They've done a complete about-face on supplements, eggs, fat: been totally discredited. The trials are warped, biased or conducted on such a small scale they're meaningless. They're taken out of context, misrepresented, sponsored by companies, even government departments, or simply made up.'

'Why?'

'To sell food or magazines, or to bullshit us into behaving the way they want us to.'

'So what *is* true then?'

'Well, cutting down on carbs seems to work, for George and me.'

'You're saying science is a lie? Medicine "wrong"?' Penelope scoffed. 'You'll claim smoking clears the tubes next.'

'No. I concede smoking's not good for you: harmful.'

'But you refuse to give up?'

'I don't want to.'

'The truth is you *can't*. It's *that* insidious, *that* dangerous. It should be *completely* illegal! And yet *you*,' she swung round to point at Reggie, 'are promoting it in hospitals. As if the patients weren't ill enough already.' The papers were now championing

168

Reggie's 'baccy bunkers' initiative, if only to bait the Health Secretary. One had even dubbed them 'the People's Pavilions'.

'Despite the fact that it is *not* illegal, smokers are already treated like criminals, Penelope, especially in hospital – or at least as some sort of under-class.' Reggie was damned if he would be told off at his own party. 'Even though, as you say, once you've started it's very hard to stop, especially if you're worried. Denying smokers their perfectly legal treat – one, incidentally, that pours billions into the Treasury – when they're frightened and ill, is downright cruel.'

Penelope dropped her gaze. The last thing she'd meant to do was antagonise her host. Bill had been right at the Cheesemongers' dinner. Reggie was worth noticing. It was his piffling friends she found insufferable. And besides, she had something to ask him.

The plates were cleared and Mikey tried to curl up in his seat. Sebastian helped him out of his cardboard wings. He sat up again when the curries arrived, accompanied by onion, mushroom and spinach bhajis, naan bread, fluffy white rice and salad. Sebastian slipped him a piece of naan, dipped in curry. The dog put his head on one side and forced it down in great gasping chomps.

'Isn't curry bad for dogs?' Penelope asked hopefully.

'I heard that too,' said Fleur.

'No more than humans. Depends what's in it,' said Tommy, whose weekly visit to the Star of India was set in stone. '*Kari* is just the Tamil word for sauce. It can contain whatever's handy: normally chilli, coriander, cumin and turmeric. The British hijacked it with the creation of curry powder. Instant curry was the catering Holy Grail of eighteenth-century Britain. All those company men returning from India. Every businessman in the empire was chasing it.'

'Weren't Lea and Perrins working on a formula when they came up with Worcestershire Sauce?'

'Yes, but it was so revolting they couldn't face it. Just left it to seethe and bubble in some cellar for eighteen months. By which time it was so virulent they thought, what the hell, and dashed it in a few sauces to see what happened.'

'Extraordinary.'

'Interesting what happens by mistake.'

'Surely it's past his bedtime?' pleaded Penelope, unable to concentrate on anything but Mikey's convulsive mouthing.

'He likes you,' said Tommy. 'He's half bulldog you know, with the soul of a Labrador. The boys'll come and fetch him in a minute.'

'I wondered why he was so ugly.'

'There ought to be a law against it, eh, Penelope?'

'You can sneer all you like, Sebastian, but as long as there are people who won't help themselves, people like you, the government is duty-bound to nudge them in the right direction.'

'Banning things without cutting off supply just makes people dig in their heels. I was always being *told* to lose weight. Just pissed me off. It wasn't until I *chose* to go along with George and Reggie that I started to make real progress. People love First Eleven because they choose to join in; they're not hounded into it by some government busybody.'

170

'May I have the fizzy water, please?' Penelope said, taking a deep breath. 'It's true that private initiatives can have a unique appeal and local relevance, *and* spare the public purse. Everyone agrees First Eleven is a *very* good thing.' Reggie's expression softened. 'Not everything has to be government sponsored or controlled, but when they aren't, they're so often ill thought-through, even irrational. Take First Eleven: I mean why cricket, Reggie? As far as getting your bang for your buck goes, in terms of time, resources, even cardio, cricket is hardly ideal. Think of all that loafing about and wasted space.'

'Think of the camaraderie and memories, the smell of new-mown grass. What could be more English than a lawn? That sound, leather on willow, distant applause.'

'Rain more like,' said the colonel.

'Yes, rain too. It's our heritage. It's *their* heritage. We have to pass it on, and we might just discover a Viv Richards or Richard Hadlee in the process. Not everything can be boiled down to bangs and bucks, Penelope.'

'You're living in the wrong century, Reggie. Cricket is like the potato. If they discovered it today it wouldn't be allowed. I saw your promotional film. Charming but amateur, so amateur! And I gather you haven't even monetised your database. Do you have a sales team?'

'No.'

'Think what cold calling could achieve! The trouble with you, Reggie,' she was wagging her finger at him again, 'is that you're sentimental, uncommercial . . .'

'What used to be called a gentleman,' said the colonel. 'Not a concept the current crop of parliamentary parasites can get their heads round.'

Penelope stood up, towering over us all.

'Where are the Ladies?' she said.

'Quite,' said the colonel.

'Let me show you,' said Jane, glaring at Valentine. They left the table.

'Does anyone have the chutney?' he asked.

'I don't want to make a scene,' said Bill Table with steely affability. 'But I don't like the way you're talking to my wife.' The colonel stared at him, goggle-eyed, too stunned to intercept the passing chutney. He was bullying a woman. So much for gentleman. Bill stared back. The colonel blinked first.

'I'm sorry. You're right. Hip making me snappy.'

'Take one of these,' someone said, tossing a tube over.

'Take two,' said Fleur, popping it open.

'What are they?'

'Painkillers.'

'Certainly not.'

'Two,' said Fleur firmly. He hesitated, and complied.

Tommy's sons sneaked in and out again, carrying Mikey off to bed. Penelope returned and noted the empty wings.

'Finally gone?' she said as she sat down. 'I bet the staff are relieved. They can't have many dogs for dinner.'

'Thank you for putting up with him,' said Tommy.

'Thank you for putting up with me,' the colonel said stiffly. 'I'm sorry I was rude.'

172

'I had dog for dinner once,' said Fleur, before the colonel could retract his apology. 'In Mexico: Chihuahua with peanuts. We were mortified when we found out. Just assumed it was guinea pig.'

'Weren't pugs originally for eating?' asked Bill.

'Probably,' his wife replied. 'Though where would you start? Each end more repulsive than the other.'

'Very hard to eat dogs, horses, donkeys,' said Reggie. 'Personalities really: friends, even colleagues. That's why I can't do salami. You never know what's in it.'

'My great-grandfather ate a colleague,' said Penelope. 'Albeit a very junior one. Accidentally, of course, in taro stew. When he was Bishop of Polynesia. An eager young curate wandered off on his own. Typical, they thought, when he was late for lunch. Didn't realise he was already there. Long pig, they called it. Only clicked when a whole hand turned up. Went to trial and everything. Rather stymied his career.'

'The curate must have been mortified,' snorted the colonel. Fleur glowered at him.

'With taro you say?' said Helen, who was writing a cookbook. 'What is taro?'

'A sort of root, I think,' said Jane. 'Like a parsnip.'

'Sodden with carbs then,' said Sebastian.

'I had elephant in Africa,' the colonel said in an uncharacteristically gentle tone. 'Never been so ashamed of anything in my life.'

'I find that hard to believe,' said Penelope. The colonel let it pass.

'What were you doing in Africa?' Bill asked quickly.

'Long story. Army. Compulsory hooley. Ordered to butter up some warlord by so-called Uncle Jim. Sticky situation all round. Never again.'

'How do you eat an elephant?' Helen asked, getting out her mobile to make notes.

'A little bit at a time,' Valentine said sadly. 'A little bit at a time.'

'Talking of eating, Reggie,' said Penelope, oblivious to the mood as ever. 'Can I give you lunch in the House as my guest? Sometime soon-ish? There's something I need to ask you.'

'The House?'

'The House of Lords.'

'How very kind, Penelope. Thank you,' Reggie said.

'Can you do Thursday the second of June?'

'I'm sorry, Penelope, I can't. That's the run-up to the Colneford Show and I need to keep myself available.'

'Of course he can,' said Jane. 'The show pretty much runs itself now and I can cope for a day. He means yes, Penelope. Don't you, Reggie?'

'Yes,' he agreed. 'If you're sure, darling. Yes, please.'

'Amazing what you get offered when you lose a bit of weight,' Jane smiled, very pleased. 'Isn't it, Reggie?'

'Amazing sailors, the Polynesians,' Sebastian mused. 'Incredible journeys in flimsy canoes: vast distances with ever-diminishing supplies. That's why so many of them pile on the pounds when food is available. Only the fat-storers made it. Perhaps that's why cannibalism became acceptable, in Tonga, New Zealand,

174

et cetera: those poor chubby cabin boys wondering why they'd been asked along.'

'Did they really have cabins?' asked Fleur. 'I suppose they must have.'

'No,' said Penelope. 'What about Papua New Guinea?'

'What about it?'

'The New Guineans. Why did they practise cannibalism?'

'No idea,' Sebastian admitted. 'Bang goes that theory. But you've given me another idea for my list, Penelope. Thank you: *Cannibal Adventure* by Willard Price. I loved that book. Have I told you about my list?' But she was beckoning a waiter.

The puddings appeared, treacle tart and ice cream or fruit salad, and Sebastian took a large swig of wine, wiped his face and hands with a napkin, grimaced in apology to the table at large, and mounted the podium.

He rapped his gavel and introduced the first lot. He was witty, pushy and very effective. He knew who and where everyone was, and what they could afford, and would not give up till they had paid it.

He got double the estimate for a week on Skiathos, triple the rate for a day's shooting in Norfolk, and a thousand pounds for a beach hut in Frinton on any Saturday in June. The colonel's port, a case of Taylors 63, went for three thousand pounds.

After thirty lots he returned triumphant and flopped back in his seat. A waiter had left a treacle tart and ice cream and a full glass of beer in front of Mikey's empty chair. Without thinking, flushed with success and forehead beaded from the spotlights, Sebastian took a great draught of Mikey's lager and then a spoonful of cooling ice cream. He stood up, removed his heavy jacket, and slumped down again. Shandy slipped into the seat beside him.

'You're a natural,' she said. 'I want you for my channel.'

'Thank you,' he said. 'And thank you for taking the beach hut.'

'What's Frinton like?' she asked.

'Best beach huts in Essex,' he said. 'Let me show you.'

'With pleasure,' she said. 'Once you approve the Dolls' House deal.'

'Now that's my kind of bribery.' He mopped his forehead.

'Never less than room temperature,' she said.

'Wait till the dancing starts.'

The colonel was a good drunk, that evening. He had popped into the Spatchcock on the way to the party and then underestimated the pre-dinner cocktails on arrival. As Fleur talked and talked, he told us later, and he sipped his wine, and sipped and sipped, he felt the pain in his hip flicker and fade, and with it years of belligerence and bitterness. He was suffused with a soaring sense of reprieve, something very like hope, perhaps just co-dydramol.

Then Reggie whisked Fleur on to the dance floor just as we returned. The colonel accepted a top-up and grinned, actually grinned at us across the table.

'Looking forward to your thoughts on my manuscript, George,' he said with woozy amiability. 'Strange to think of someone reading the thing after all these years. Funny old time, the sixties. In some ways, I suppose, the best years of my life, though the world was going to hell in a hand-cart, of course, what with that frightful Kennedy and Wilson and the poor Czechs and more than one cultural revolution. It's a wonder we could sleep in our beds. Heath!'

We looked up at the sound of scraping chairs and saw Sebastian snatching a final blob of ice cream before Shandy lugged him off to dance. The colonel chuckled. 'I think my money's safe, don't you? Grace Brown's not a bad chap. Rather went up in my estimation when he tore the picture off the wall. Hee-hee-hee. Fucking Freud indeed! Hee-hee-hee. That'll teach the toerag. Well done, Brown!'

'What picture?' asked Jeremy, whose firm specialises in art insurance.

'Pinion's poxy portrait,' said the colonel, wiping tears from his eyes. 'At the Spatchcock.'

'The Spatchcock's one of ours,' Jeremy said, who was still a non-executive.

'One of your what?'

'Clients. The Freud's worth millions. What happened?' The colonel told him.

'How very alarming,' he said.

It was not many drinks later that the colonel himself asked Fleur to dance. Reggie had ditched his feathered hat, Tommy his flying helmet and the colonel his beret long ago. Now, with no pain in his hip for the first time in years, he threw off his Sam Brown too, and his tunic, and folded his arms. Half squatting, he began kicking his feet out in turn, Cossack style, faster and faster, eyes locked on Fleur, upper body still, legs figuring away like a Highland sword dancer. Fleur floated round him like a white moth, her pleated Egyptian dress billowing, arms and hands twisting and swirling, eyes lowered. When the next song started they returned, breathless and laughing.

'Time to leave,' she said. ' I can't top that. What a tremendous evening.'

It was only a few hundred yards to the Farmers' Club but heavy rain made walking unthinkable, so Fleur accepted a lift from Shandy, who murmured into her mobile to summon Peter. Within seconds the Bentley was outside.

The colonel cloaked Fleur in her mink and then gallantly held up his duffel coat, like a canopy, but an umbrella blossomed at the side of the car and Peter dashed up through the deluge to take her across. As he shut the door his umbrella blew inside out, and the colonel proffered his duffel coat again, matador style, for Shandy. She backed into the folds, clutched them around herself, pulling the hood right down over her head, and darted into the rain. Peter slammed her door, then his, and the car slicked off into the night.

'This is the best party I've been to in years,' said the colonel, shrugging his tunic back on. 'Did you see Pinion bidding for my port? Little shit. I'll give him health and safety. Let's pop round to the Spatchcock and deal with that fucking portrait once and for all.'

178

CHAPTER 7

'There must be a beginning to any great matter but it is
the continuing unto the end until it be thoroughly
finished that yields the true glory.'
　　　Sir Francis Drake, Dispatch to Walsingham 1587

'Stay me with flagons, comfort me with apples.'
　　　The Song of Solomon, 2:5, *The King James Bible*

Though it was a Saturday and nearing the end of the academic
year, it was still term time and the whole university was locked
down for exams. Sebastian's daughter Natasha had insisted on a
wedding at least six weeks before the baby was due and, as they
were both graduates, the couple had a double claim on a service
in their old College Chapel. Noise and numbers were restricted,
however, as finals were in full swing, and the party afterwards, a
late picnic lunch, was to be way outside the town towards
Grantchester, on the banks of the River Cam.

Since the New Year, we three dieters had been working towards
the vague deadline of 'when filming starts'. The production

company had now finally confirmed it would begin on Monday 13 June and the end was suddenly in sight. At our latest weigh-in that Thursday, Reggie had lost five pounds, Sebastian had lost one and I had lost two. We agreed that the next weigh-in would be no later than the first week of June, by which time, it seemed clear, Reggie would be more than camera ready.

Sebastian had organised a bus to collect the picnic and the wedding guests staying with family and friends in Essex and to get us to the College Chapel by eleven thirty. It duly dropped us on King's Parade and we made our way past the Senate House to the College in mellow May sunshine. Sebastian and Natasha arrived by flower-bedecked punt, expertly poled downriver by Natasha's old roommate.

The service was as simple and beautiful as the Chapel and, after photographs on the bridge, the bride and groom settled back into their cushions and were ferried smoothly upstream by Milo's best man, languid and lugubrious in a frock coat and top hat. The rest of us walked or took the bus the few hundred yards to Mill Lane, just above the weir, where Sebastian had reserved twenty-five punts. We stowed our coats and ties in the bus and transferred the picnic to the quay. Eight of Milo's friends stripped off their shoes, socks and trousers and – when the marital punt arrived – shunted it and its newlywed cargo over the weir slide to the upper part of the river.

Sebastian strode from punt to punt, checking each had a pole, a paddle and four cushions, and doling out bottles and glasses. The bulk of the picnic hampers and cold boxes were loaded into his, of which he insisted on taking sole charge. At first people hopped or lurched from one flat-bottomed boat – barely more than a floating tray – to another, trying to fill or pass glasses, settling into seats then changing their minds, or attempting to cast off and get out of the way, but gradually the chaos began to subside. Once each craft had four or five passengers and someone with a pole at the back, Sebastian urged them off out into the current, leaving him alone still moored to the quay.

'You need to make some room, Sebo,' Mary shouted from mid-river. 'Natasha and I asked your American friend. Apparently you've been getting on like a house on fire.'

'What? Shandy's coming?'

'She's got a meeting round the corner but promised to make it. Just texted to say she's on her way.'

Sebastian's punt was already over-laden, and he gazed down at the jumble of boxes, bottles and hampers, for once quite clearly flummoxed. There was certainly no sitting room.

The blue Bentley pulled up to the railings and Shandy jumped out and waved her floppy straw hat.

'Over here, Shandy,' Sebastian bawled, waving back. 'Through the gate. How good to see you! Just give me a second to clear a space.' He bent and scrabbled ineffectually at the boxes and baskets until Shandy arrived, tossed in her shoes and put her arms round his pot-belly from behind. Turning he kissed her, standing on tiptoe, and she kissed him back.

'You know what the Cheesemongers say?' said Jane loudly.

'What?' said Sebastian.

'When baiting the trap with cheese, always leave room for the mouse.'

'I have an awful feeling you're the mouse, Shandy,' Sebastian said, looking down at his cargo and scratching his head.

'Does that make you the cheese?' she replied, giving him another kiss. 'I'll stand with you at the back. You can teach me.'

'Deal.' He beamed, grabbing a pole and jumping onto the platform at the stern. He held out a hand. 'Stand here between my arms.' She looked down to find her footing and stepped aboard. A boatman released the punt and threw the chain on board. Sebastian pushed off.

Someone started clapping, others joined in, and soon everyone was cheering, laughing and whistling.

'Where've you been?' he asked, laughing too and struggling slightly to get the boat pointing up river.

'Lunch at the Fitzwilliam.'

'The museum. Why?'

'Treasures. Things we think our viewers would appreciate.'

'How'd it go?'

'They were . . . hard to read.'

'I'm sorry if they were difficult.'

'More obtuse than difficult: a cultural thing, I guess. I'll get the hang of it.'

'Of course you will.'

'But any assistance gratefully received. It would be fun, you know?'

'I'm beginning to think it might. Have you seen our redraft?'

'Seen it? I've gone through it line by line, word by word. Those dolls' houses better be worth it. You know my guys call you "the problem"?'

'I'm just watching my friend's back.'

'I know. Anyway, they've agreed. I'm not saying they're happy, but it's a deal.'

'A big yes! Reggie will be thrilled.'

'I am,' shouted Reggie from a neighbouring punt. 'I *am*!'

'If the supply ship is quite ready,' Fleur chirruped. 'Shall we set sail?'

The lead punts, just holding their own against the gentle current till now, nosed out into midstream and set off towards the open countryside, the banks getting wilder and more unkempt as we slipped out of town. We passed under bridges of various types and sizes, until the last, a massive concrete lintel with a road thundering overhead proved the gateway to proper fields dotted with black and white cows.

There were no footpaths here and few other punts. The recent graduates and post-graduates, those most familiar with the vagaries of the river, took the lead, warning the rest of us of the sudden depths, where the bottom was out of reach, or the patches of mud that could grip a pole, tricking punters into yanking themselves in as they determinedly clung on and their boats slid out from under them. The sun warmed our shirts. Rafts of duck squabbled in our wake, alert for titbits, and we nudged through families of swans, gawky grey cygnets milling within their parents' charge; tense white adults quivering with menace.

Reggie and I had a punt each. Like Sebastian we had rolled up our sleeves, shed our shoes and socks and shaken out our rusty skills. I remembered myself as deft and fast, but it was all I could do now to keep up.

Sebastian's punt swooshed between us, water chuckling down its sides. Shandy had the pole now, with Sebastian behind her, one arm round her waist. They edged ahead.

'Come on, slowcoaches,' he mocked. We lunged after them in silent parallel, working too hard to talk, following the armada into a long, shallower stretch flanked by woods. Bright green dragonflies hovered and darted alongside, large fish lolled in the sunlit depths. We turned into a sharp corner, cleared the trees, and were back in the open again, within tinny earshot of a jazz quartet, tootling away beneath an awning hanging from a blasted willow.

A convoy of bemused Japanese were watching the band in astonishment, their punts straddling the waterway, mystified by the solitary performance in the middle of nowhere. Our arrival provided an answer and they raised their telephones in unison to photograph the wedding punt, its top-hatted captain, and the flotilla in its wake. Some tried to clear us a passage using their punt poles as oars, tightening the gridlock. Shandy thanked them in cheerful Japanese and they laughed delightedly.

'Show off,' said Sebastian proudly. He clambered round her and on to the picnic, rummaging about at the sides for the paddle. He drew it out like Excalibur and brandished it two handed, slicing the air, Samurai style. The tourists took his photograph but made no move to find their own oars, so he knelt on the boxes and mimed paddling to the side. This did the trick and, following his lead, they floundered to the water iris at the banks, allowing us to pass.

A few yards later we turned in to join the musicians, passengers hopping ashore to secure the boats with chains and spikes. As more and more arrived, rugs were spread out on the grass and folding chairs and cushions deployed. The band were plied with praise and drink. Sebastian brought his craft in broadside; the boxes and baskets were heaved on to the turf and flung open by the strongest or greediest members of the party. We pulled in behind him to the sound of popping corks, tinkling glasses, the drum, sax, horn and clarinet.

After years of preparing the mid-morning shoot drinks, there is no better picnicker than Sebastian and, as ever, he had doubled what twice our number could reasonably be expected to eat and drink.

'Talk about well catered for,' said Fleur. 'You've gone completely over the top as usual, Sebo. Where's my chair?' He opened out a cluster of four folding chairs and set two empty cold boxes in front of her as a table. Three elderly sisters came over to join her. Sebastian gave them drinks.

'Food is like money, Fleur,' said Tommy. 'Only too much is enough.' He fired a champagne cork into the river and handed the bottle to Sebastian who dived into the throng, filling glasses right and left. Mary beckoned us over and we flopped down beside her on a pile of punt cushions.

'Please let it work out between Shandy and Sebo,' she sighed. 'I'd so love him to be happy . . . and off my hands.'

'He's been off your hands for yonks, Mary,' Fiona said.

'He's like glandular fever . . . he can linger for years. Anyway, he's such a blundering teddy bear. On days like today I just want

185

to take him home and give him a cuddle.' She slowly sipped her champagne, watching Sebastian sort out more folding chairs for yet more aged relations. 'Then I actually talk to him and remember why we split in the first place.' She watched as he bounced over to Shandy and some of Natasha's friends. 'I mean, the rows we had about these bloody champagne glasses! He insisted on these flat jobs, even though the tall ones, what are they called?'

'Flutes.'

'Exactly. Even though these take up ten times more room than the flute ones and are incredibly fragile. The champagne doesn't taste any different.'

'Are you becoming an old bag, Mary?' said Tommy. 'Are you all right?'

'Not sure.'

Sebastian said something to Shandy that made everybody laugh.

'She is good news,' said Fiona.

'Have you googled her?' Mary asked Fiona.

'Of course,' Fiona admitted. 'Rich as Croesus, hugely successful, and widowed.'

'I know. And beautiful, the bitch! I just assumed she was divorced.'

'Husband was obviously some sort of genius.'

'Can someone get me another chair?' Fleur demanded, tottering over. 'Sebo parked me with the old farts.' I found a chair and opened it out for her.

'Physicist. Brilliant, but had a stroke: four years in a coma till they switched him off five years ago.'

'Awful,' said Fiona. 'Poor Shandy.'

'Who are you talking about?' Fleur demanded.

'Shandy's husband.'

'What about him?'

'He's dead.'

'Dear Sebo,' said Fleur. 'I hope he knows what he's getting into.'

'I hope *she* knows what she's getting into,' said Mary. 'I don't want her handing him back.'

'A scholar, a sweetie pie,' said Fleur. 'And a Grace Brown. What more could you ask?'

'The girls adored him when we first hit London,' said Tommy.

'None more than me!' said Mary. 'I was . . . whatever it's called: love struck. God, he was gorgeous! And a sensational snogger.'

'Erotic technique,' said Tommy. 'You've either got it or you haven't.'

'Screw erotic technique,' said Fleur. 'All girls want is kindness, keenness and cash.'

'Well, he can certainly be keen,' said Mary. 'And kind.'

'And she's got the cash,' said Tommy.

'I'm not sure he'd necessarily like that,' said Mary.

'Don't be ridiculous!' said Fleur.

Holding a bottle of Sancerre, Sebastian picked his way back through his recumbent guests, found himself an empty glass, grabbed a chair and slumped into it next to Fleur.

'Hello Auntie,' he said, clinking his glass on hers. 'Anyone seen Shandy? Thank you so much for asking her, Mary. She was with me two seconds ago.'

'She's chatting up Milo's parents. Everyone adores her. Having fun?'

'I am.' He took a sip. 'And I've just had some rather good news.'

'We heard. The Dolls' House deal.'

'Not that.'

'What then?'

'Shandy's read the colonel's manuscript and loves it.'

'What colonel?'

'My colonel,' said Fleur.

'Colonel Derek. Valentine Derek, old friend of Reggie's, new friend of Fleur's, member of the Spatchcock, has written a book. Or at least wrote one years ago. He lent Shandy his coat with the manuscript in the pocket. Shandy says it's brilliant.'

'What's it called?'

'*It's All About Mimi.*'

'What?'

'It's all about Mimi: Princess Mimi. Valentine was the dashing young "conducting officer" to the daughter of Hal Jackhammer, the American armaments guy, over in London being schmoozed by the MOD. Mimi Jackhammer was twenty-one and the apple of her father's eye. Valentine was deputised to show her the sights. He took her everywhere that was anywhere in sixties London: shops, clubs, restaurants, galleries and shows. Access and money no object.'

'What fun.'

'Terrific fun. But after a while, of course, she and her father returned home, and several years later she married Prince Nog

188

of Moldova and became Emelia Moldova. Princess Mimi: American royalty. A modern-day Grace Kelly. Shandy has snapped up the book and film rights and is going to build a London tour around it.'

'What does Princess Mimi say? She's still alive, isn't she? And rather glam.'

'Gave her blessing to the manuscript years ago. Valentine submitted it for her approval when he first wrote it.'

'He would,' said Fleur. 'That's so Valentine.'

'Shandy spoke to her last week and she's offered to put her name to the introduction.'

'What does Valentine say?' Fleur asked, rubbing her hands.

'Over the moon, apparently. Looking forward to spending his advance . . . on you.'

'I wish you'd asked him today, Sebo,' said Fleur.

'Sorry, Fleur. Numbers a bit tight.'

'Well, I just hope Reggie doesn't think like that when he's . . . you know.'

'What do you mean?'

'You were there, Sebo, when Penelope Table asked him to lunch at the House of Lords.'

'So?'

'She's a cabinet minister with responsibility for "Health and Wellbeing". He's a kind and successful businessman, as honest as the day is long, who's never done a mean thing in his life. A lovely family man and brilliant philanthropist, who has just lost a fifth of his body weight and is about to feature in a documentary about a charity he founded – and pretty much pays for – that

189

introduces children to our national sport. Talk about health and wellbeing! Why would she be asking him to the House of Lords? If he isn't noble, I don't know who is.'

'You're right, Fleur. Yet more good news! What an incredible day! Good old Penny!'

'Do you think he has any idea?'

'Not sure, but I think Jane has. She'd make the perfect Lady Lambert.'

Mary picked up an empty champagne bottle and put it down. Sebastian popped out of his chair, found a full bottle, filled her glass and lolled back down again.

'I was just saying, Sebo, what an incredible fuss you made about the glasses,' Mary said, holding up her drink and looking at the sun through the bubbles. 'Is it because they were moulded from Marie Antoinette's left breast or something?'

'No. It's because my mother loved them. And they had nothing to do with poor Marie Antoinette's left breast. That's just vile French propaganda: revolutionary, anti-monarchist, republican propaganda.'

'If you say so, darling.'

'The design was created by Venetian glass blowers in the early 1660s, in London, at least ninety years before her birth. It's the hideous flute jobs that are a French design: eighteenth-century Parisian.'

'But you're having Sancerre, Sebo. What's up?'

'Carbs.'

'I thought champagne had the same amount of calories as normal wine? Roughly 120 a glass.'

'A few more in champagne, I think. But a glass of white wine has about one gram of carbs, red has a half, and fizzy wine six.'

'So you're having six times the amount of Sancerre.'

'Yes.'

'Don't get too pissed before the speeches,' Mary told him.

'Why not?' He laughed. 'On today of all days? I'm not even making a speech.'

'Sorry. None of my beeswax. I feel like I'm being orphaned or something. Things coming to an end.'

'Beginning more like: grandchildren!'

'God. I'll be a granny!'

'I tell you what *is* coming to an end. You've just made up my mind: this frightful diet.' He noticed a pork pie on a plate, cut it into three unequal slices, smothered the largest piece in English mustard, dipped it in mayonnaise and ate it.

Mary propped herself up in alarm.

'What are you talking about, Sebo? You've got nowhere yet.'

'What do you mean nowhere? I've lost sixteen pounds. You try picking up thirty-two pats of butter. But I've been on it for months and months and I'm fed up. Or fed down. We've done the wedding photographs and Shandy doesn't give a hoot what I look like. It's time to boot it into touch.'

'Remember what Hank said.'

'Hank can bugger off, talking of beeswax. We were doing it for Reggie, weren't we, George? And he's more than camera ready. Quite fancy him myself.'

'I'll talk to Shandy.'

'Don't you dare, Mary!'

191

Reggie stood, pulled his morning coat back on, tinkled a knife against a bottle and began his speech. He was touching and funny about Natasha for fifteen minutes, toasted her and sat down.

Milo took his place, agreed with him about Natasha. Thanked the band, college, chaplain, florists, dress-maker, punters, Sebastian and Mary, his own parents, friends and Natasha, even the Japanese, and promised to be the best possible husband and father. On behalf of them both he then thanked Reggie and me for helping Sebastian through 'his scare'. Only Sebastian could have made so light of 'such an awful scare', he said, and come through it unscathed.

'Enough of that,' said Sebastian, raising his glass like an Olympic torch. He saw Shandy looking puzzled and grinned at her.

'We're just so grateful you're here, Daddy . . . Still with us.' Natasha gulped.

The best man, still in his top hat and frock coat, then launched into a series of mystifying magic tricks while making his speech, illustrating Milo's life and courtship with twisty balloons, coloured handkerchiefs and a rabbit. He had a doctorate in anthropology and lectured on primitive magic. Finally he swept off his stovepipe topper, releasing a pair of doves, pink and blue, slammed the hat down on a picnic hamper and waved his magic wand.

'Abracadabra!' we all shouted. He whipped away the hat to reveal a three-tiered wedding cake and we stood to toast the bridesmaids.

Sebastian and Mary walked over to the riverbank to stand with the bride and groom for the cutting of the cake. After the photographs, with the Japanese trying to turn their punts in the background, having all now shipped their poles and resorted to paddles, people began returning to their seats or finding new ones.

'What a brilliant magician!' raved Fleur. 'And what a sweet little cake. Like a white telescope. Has it been in his hat all this time? Amazing it didn't disintegrate, especially when he banged it down like that.'

'Incredibly strong, wedding cakes,' said Reggie. 'You know St Bride's on Fleet Street? The Cheesemongers' chapel?'

'You mean the journalists' chapel?' she said.

'We were there first. Centuries earlier,' Reggie insisted. 'Anyway, when Thomas Rich, an apprentice baker working opposite on Ludgate Hill, just below St Paul's, finally got permission to marry his master's daughter, he decided to make the cake for his wedding in the image of St Bride's, where they were due to be married, which had burnt down in the Fire of London and just been rebuilt by Christopher Wren.'

'When was this?'

'About 1700. Anyway Rich's cake, which became the talk of London, needed such thick icing to hold up all those tiers that it took the two of them, bride and groom, holding the knife together, to actually cut the thing, starting the modern tradition.'

'What a charming story,' said Fleur. 'So we have something else to thank the Cheesemongers for.'

'Is Shandy all right?' Reggie said, noticing Shandy making her way towards Sebastian, negotiating bodies, rugs and cushions, no longer smiling now, looking solemn and perplexed. He intercepted her and brought her over.

'Are you okay, Shandy?'

'Is Sebo okay? What's this scare? This awful scare?'

'Has he not mentioned it?' asked Fleur.

'What?'

'His heart attack. Ages ago. Valentine's Day. He's fine now.'

Without a word, Shandy left, crossing to Sebastian and then hovering behind him. He was still laughing and joking with the bride and groom and Milo's parents. He clapped Milo on the shoulder and turned to face her, enfolding her in a slightly tipsy bear hug, before taking her hand and dragging her back over.

'What's this scare, Sebo?' we could hear her asking. 'Are you okay?'

'Of course I am. I overdid it, that's all. Months ago. Look, here comes the cake.'

'But you said you were great.'

'I *am* great!' He hugged her again. 'And so are you.'

Emily, his other daughter, handed us each a tiny piece of wedding cake in a Bakelite bowl. Someone else, rather drunk, was reluctantly bestowing strawberries, one at a time, on the waiting crowd. A girl in a bikini and a droopy sombrero was dispensing cream and ice cream.

'What do the doctors say?' persisted Shandy.

'It was a one-off.' Sebastian accepted large portions of everything on top of the cake.

'So you did have a heart attack? Why didn't you tell me?'

'Because I'm fine. Didn't seem relevant. Didn't want to put you off. Just a bit more ice cream, please. Yes. Yes . . . And brown sugar, please . . . Perfect . . . And then cream on top, please. Have you seen this, Shandy? I love the way the cream holds the sugar when it freezes on the ice cream. Are you not having any?' He looked round for a seat. She fumbled in her handbag and the ringtone sounded, distant trumpets. She took it out and switched it off.

'Sebastian,' she said gravely, standing up straight all of a sudden. He looked up at her, smiling. She stooped and kissed his shiny pink forehead. 'Sorry.'

'What for?'

'I have to brief the guys on the Fitzwilliam thing. Got to go. Will you thank Mary and Natasha for me? I've had . . . It's been awesome. I'll hitch a ride with the Japanese. They could use a pilot, even a novice. Thanks for the lesson. Peter's waiting.' She reached the bank in a few strides and stepped straight off onto the back of a Japanese punt, picking up a pole as she did so. The passengers wailed as it dipped several inches and then bobbed back up again. She plunged her pole into the water and pushed off with one giant thrust. 'I had . . . a good time.'

'Bye,' Sebastian shouted cheerfully. 'Talk later.'

She shoved out into midstream and lunged back towards the town, with the current this time, leaving the remaining Japanese calling vainly after their friends.

'What was that all about?' demanded Fleur.

195

'If it's not a big yes . . .?' said Tommy.

'Isn't she adorable?' sighed Sebastian.

Reggie is President of the Colneford Show and almost single-handedly responsible for its survival. On buying the big house in 1990 and learning that the village green had been denied insurance, he instantly called Jeremy at Lloyd's, set up a local action group, and offered his own garden and adjacent fields as an alternative showground in the meanwhile. Within a week it was an annual commitment.

He quickly restored the cricket match. There had always been a dog show, so it seemed only natural to invite livestock back, first poultry and ponies, then goats, then sheep, cows, pigs and now even alpacas. In due course, with support from the Cheesemongers, a cheese tent was introduced. Flowers, vegetables, cakes and jams were old favourites, but soon ploughing and vintage vehicles were added, and steam pumps.

On the retirement of his predecessor, Reggie was the obvious choice for president, and tea in the President's Tent, one of his mobile cricket pavilions, became one of the most sought-after invitations in northeast Essex. Shops, stalls and sponsors became involved, in a modest way, and the week before the show, horseboxes, trucks and caravans began to converge on what had become known as Royal Colneford. This year was to be the best attended ever and Reggie was rushed off his feet. Nevertheless, he insisted we snatch a quick weigh-in on the Saturday morning.

'I'm sorry to have to tell you,' he said when we walked through his kitchen door, 'that they've cancelled the documentary.'

'What unutterable wankers,' said Sebastian. 'After you put yourself through hell. Why?'

'Doing something on English sparkling wine instead.'

'Can they do that?'

'They can do what they like. Very disappointing for the whole team at First Eleven, of course, but to be honest . . . I'm rather relieved.'

'You don't look it. You look miserable. Didn't you have a contract or something? I thought you were a businessman?'

'I'm retired.'

'Well, I've ditched the diet anyway. Forget the scales.'

'Certainly not, Sebo. Aren't you at least curious to see what you weigh? And what about the colonel?'

'Talking of pounds of flesh. He's such a ferocious old fart.' Sebastian glowered at the dark plastic square in the middle of the floor. 'All right, then. Though I bet you a tenner you've already weighed yourself?'

'Of course.'

'Out with it then.' For an answer, Reggie flipped off his shoes and stepped gingerly on to the scales: thirteen stone thirteen pounds. 'Three and a half stone down!'

'You've done it, Reggie!' I said. 'You've done it!'

'Wouldn't have happened without you two. Thank you. I really am grateful.'

'And how's the pre-diabetes?'

'Gone. As soon as I lost that first stone.'

'Smug bastard,' muttered Sebastian. 'Has it occurred to you that they cancelled the documentary because you no longer look the part? Perhaps they *wanted* a pregnant bulldog? Fat cats are two a penny.'

'Couldn't go on as I was. It wasn't just the way I looked. I felt sort of clogged by all that bulk; trapped. I feel infinitely better now.'

'Good,' Sebastian replied. 'So we can start eating again. Much has been lost. Much is to be regained! They've got everything out there: biscuits, cake.' He rubbed his hands. 'Pam's fudge. I presume she won again?' Reggie nodded. 'Of course she did,' continued Sebastian. 'What a heroine.'

'But I thought you were the judge?' I said.

'Of the fudge? Not any more: dumped. They suddenly decided I was biased, after seven years, because Pam works for my aunt. They've put me on the cider instead. Later today.'

'Oh God, Sebo, I'd forgotten about that. Please be ... careful.'

'Only if *you* promise *not* to be careful,' Sebastian replied. 'And come off that bloody diet and start eating properly again.'

'No. I refuse to go bonkers and put it all back on. I will start eating properly ... but only for five days a week.'

'What?'

'I'm going on the Fast Diet.'

'But you've done it, you bozo. You've got there! The weight's off. The telly's off. Surely the diet's off?'

'I like being thinner and fitter, Sebo. I'm not going back.'

'Poof,' said Sebastian.

'Though I am looking forward to drinking again. A whopping great pint!'

'Several,' said Sebastian.

198

'Can you remember breakfast in the Cock and Bull when I was so outraged by the way you were packing your face? And you said you were on the Fast Diet and it was perfectly okay?'

'Of course I remember. It was totally useless. I hardly lost a pound!'

'But you did! Between our first lunch in the Spatchcock and our Valentine's weigh-in you ate like a pig . . . for five days a week! And look at our sheet.' Reggie smoothed down the page. 'You didn't lose *a* pound, you lost *four*. But the main point is you didn't *gain* anything! And I saw how much you were eating . . . for weeks. It defied reason, but it worked. So I'm going on the Fast Diet too . . . for ever!' Sebastian and I exchanged looks. 'Mondays and Thursdays.' Reggie nudged the scales with his toe. 'Come on. Let's see how you've done.'

Without bothering to take off his jacket or shoes, Sebastian stepped on the scales. Reggie stooped to examine the green digital display.

'Blimey, Sebo,' he said. 'Would you mind just stepping off and then on again? It doesn't compute.' Sebastian did as instructed. Reggie bowed over the read-out, hands on knees, and then straightened up. 'No. That's what it says. In less than three weeks since our last weigh-in, you've *put on* eighteen pounds!' He picked our sheet off the table. 'After five months of non-stop dieting, you've *gained* two pounds. What have you been doing?'

'Comfort eating.'

'But what about your heart?'

'You mean Shandy?'

'No, your *heart* heart.'

'Fuck that. You heard about the message?' We both nodded. Of course we had. The morning after the wedding, Shandy had ended their relationship, by voicemail. 'She's vanished. Won't answer her mobile. I just get your bloody Ludo, George, if I call her work number, who's now – what do they call it – her gate-keeper.' He shook his head. 'And he's taking the piss. He puts on a sort of singsong corporate voice. "I'm sorry, caller, Ms Madison is not available right now."'

'He doesn't really call you caller?'

'No. But he does use a robot voice.'

'You're being unfair.'

'Of course. I'm hacked off and . . . sad . . . I suppose.'

'It was hearing about your heart attack that did it, after all she'd been through with her husband. She didn't want to get close to someone else who might . . . It's a sort of compliment really.'

'Tommy said she thinks I was bullshitting her.'

'You were,' Reggie said. 'You should have told her. I'm sorry, Sebo.'

'When, Reggie? When should I have told her? It would've been pathetic: "I've had a heart attack, but will you go out with me anyway?"' Reggie blew his nose. 'Exactly,' said Sebastian. 'But the upside is, I have no reason not to get eating and drinking now it's all over, and smoking for Britain: fine wine, food and fags.'

'Don't tell me: the three *f*s. And of course grandchildren don't really need grandfathers,' Reggie said, suddenly angry. 'It's the

grannies that make the real difference. Everybody knows that!'
He held out his hand for my jacket. 'Your turn, George.'

I had lost a pound.

'*Almost* three stone, George,' he said, writing the figures on
our sheet. 'Four more pounds to reach your target and then that
extra five for good measure. Nine pounds in all.' He stepped
back and looked me up and down. 'Two months if you pull your
finger out.'

'*Two months?*' said Sebastian. 'Too long.'

I wasn't thin, in fact I was still overweight, but I wasn't really
fat any more either. The snoring had stopped at thirteen stone
ten pounds, and instead of my sons pinching my clothes, I was
borrowing theirs, occasionally, and digging out some of my own
that had been consigned to the mothballs years ago. But there
was a fiftieth coming up and a holiday . . . and then I remembered
that bolt of tweed in Savile Row.

'A doddle,' I said. 'Walk in the park.'

Jane clattered in, dressed for a Buckingham Palace garden
party, in enormous cream hat, matching jacket, skirt and shoes.

'Hello darling,' said Reggie. 'Do you think those heels are
quite right for grass?'

'Reggie!' she snapped. 'Where's your tie? We're due at Jerry's
pig-out at twelve.'

'Sorry, darling.' He quickly put on a jacket and tie and picked
up his battered panama. She hurried out ahead of us, tutting.

'What's up with Jane?' Sebastian asked. 'She didn't even say
hello.'

'I left her to hold the fort yesterday. She's a bit pissed off.'

'Why?'

'Lunch with Penelope Table, in London.'

'In the House of Lords. Have you had that already? You sneaky bastard. You could have told us.'

'Didn't think you'd be interested.'

'So no news then?'

'No.'

'Oh, don't tell me you turned it down, Reggie? No wonder Jane's baity.'

'Of course I didn't turn it down. I like the guy.'

'Sorry, what are we talking about?'

'Her husband, Bill. Penny asked me to help him into the Spatchcock.'

'What?'

'She still feels guilty about the "top and side Table" comments. Thinks he needs somewhere of his own now they work together. A sort of sanctuary.'

'Of course he does: from her! I am sorry, Reggie. That *and* the documentary. No wonder Jane's so down in the dumps.'

'The good news is that Fat Jack's back in the hall at the Spatchcock, as dogged and doughty as ever.'

'That *is* good news,' said Sebastian. 'Though I haven't managed to get there recently.'

'Jerry's firm heard rumours of late-night shenanigans on the premises, drunken brawls, gratuitous vandalism, and felt unable to insure the portrait after all. And of course that put the wind up all the other insurers.'

'Understandably.'

'And the committee could never hang it uninsured.'

'Of course not. It's one of Freud's largest.'

'So out went Pinion and back came Jack.'

'Are you lot coming?' Jane yelled from the garden. 'Or shall I go on my own?'

Jeremy's organic Essex saddleback pork was the best organic Essex saddleback pork any of us had ever tasted, and crackling was carb free. We set off through the garden towards the show.

Not only had one of Jeremy's sows won first prize, but his chipolatas were to be featured in *The Five Colnes Gazette*, and he had laid on a gigantic spit as well as his signature sweet-and-sour pork in celebration.

Reggie and Jane joined Jeremy in front of the Porkmobile, an old kebab van painted like a saddleback pig. Sebastian and I stood with Fiona in the audience. Jeremy's own insurance company generously donated the silver champion's cup a few years ago, and he passed it to Reggie so that he could be photographed giving it back to him, as happened every year. Though the van had clearly been doing a roaring trade for some time, Reggie then formally declared it open and the scramble for orders resumed.

People were reeling away from the counter with large punnets of rice topped with succulent chunks of pale pork, drenched in amber goo, the sweat bursting from their foreheads and upper lips in reaction to the zip in the sauce, but still chopsticking away with yelps of appreciation. After a few token mouthfuls and a splinter of crackling, Sebastian peeled off towards the cider tent and Fiona and I went on general walkabout. We tried on ponchos and bought some chutney, patted cows and fondled lambs.

Between the goats and the lawnmowers, Reggie had somehow persuaded Porsche to take a stand. Fiona sat in the lowest and reddest, with and without its roof, and wondered out loud if we might get it on tick. The salesman gave me his card. I clasped my hands behind my back and leant against the railings and a goat gently nibbled it from my grasp.

We watched a cousin almost win the ploughing competition. Then Fiona received a text to say that one of her godchildren was due in to bat and we made our way to the edge of the cricket pitch, where his proud parents had set out deckchairs and were hurriedly doling out Pimm's before he reached the crease. By three forty-five he had scored 21 very cautious runs. We congratulated his parents and headed for the President's Tent.

Reggie's most magnificent portable cricket pavilion sat right in the middle of the showground, on the edge of the parade ring, with veranda and sunny enclosure marked off by a miniature white picket fence. A thirty-foot pennant emblazoned with 'The President's Tent' fluttered above it, and stewards in bowler hats stood on either side of the entrance.

After they had been formally scrutinised we were given back our invitations and nodded through into a large room lined with benches and lockers. A row of trestle tables piled with cakes, sandwiches, biscuits, glasses, plates, saucers and tea cups was manned by women in matching aprons, wielding jugs of orange squash and brown tin teapots. I recognised Pam and June. Reggie was helping three white-coated cowmen to plates of cake.

One wall opened right out on to the veranda, the enclosure and – beyond the low picket fence – the show ring.

Sebastian accepted a cup of tea from Pam, while sizing up the cakes, and absentmindedly added four sugars, neatly sidestepping a small glass bucket and two bulbous bottles at his feet: one full of weak coffee, apparently, and the other with what looked like toadstools in vinegar.

'More Victoria sponge coming in a minute,' Pam assured him. 'I'll bring you a slice. Shall I look after the cider for you? And the pickled apples? Get them out of the way. And your beautiful presentation cup?'

'Thank you,' he said, passing the glass bucket, the cider cup.

'How was it? The cider show, I mean?'

'Super, Pam, thank you,' he said solemnly, heaving the bottles across the table. She stowed them under the tablecloth. 'Very, very good. It took ages to plump on the winner: hardly a hairsbreadth in it. And then the Essex cider makers very kindly gave me the pickled apples and that lovely flagon cider cup.'

'It is a beauty.'

'A flagon is two pints.'

'Is it?' she said, holding it up to the light. It was engraved with apple blossom.

'And the judges always get a flagon of the winning cider to take home.' He smiled at her soppily. She scowled. 'Though I'd much rather have fudge, of course.'

'All's well that ends well,' she said, putting the glass with the flagons.

'Congratulations, as ever, Pam, on your victory. Did you save me my usual? Fleur gave you the dosh?'

'Not much doubt about the fudge champion this year, I'm pleased to say. I left your order by the yard door for when you leave.'

'Thank you, Pam. My friends can't get enough. I might pop back to the sweetie tent and snaffle a mini bag now.'

'Sold out in the tent I'm afraid, Sebastian, but I may have something in my baskets round the back. I'll have a look for you when I get a moment.'

A pack of foxhounds entered the ring, with the Mistress on a skewbald Connemara, and then some boisterous bassets presided over by a fat man on foot in velvet hunting cap, pink coat, britches and black rugby boots. He tooted his horn.

'Isn't that Geoffrey Bramley?' Sebastian asked. 'Who was going to diet with us?'

'Yes,' agreed Reggie, helping himself to a cup of tea. 'Got too heavy to keep up with his hounds.'

'So he lost the weight on his own?' asked Jane. 'He was enormous I remember.'

'Didn't lose an ounce. Switched from beagles to bassets: lower and slower. Gave his beagles to the Trinity Foot and adopted that pack from Suffolk. They're about half the speed, apparently. Still has visiting rights with the beagles, of course, and a free sub.'

'Jane?' said a strident voice.

'Lambert?' growled another: Valentine and Fleur. 'I see the diet's been abandoned,' said the colonel, eyeing the massive slice of Victoria sponge on Sebastian's plate. 'What's the tally? There's quite a serious book running on these results back at the Spatchcock. I wouldn't be at all surprised if I was in the money.'

'You are,' said Reggie. 'By twenty pounds.' He took the Spatchcock sheet out of his pocket and handed it over.

'Twenty pounds?' Valentine hooked his walking stick over his left arm and brought the sheet up to his eyes. 'Only twenty?' He looked suspiciously at Sebastian, who was now discreetly licking the jam and cream from his fingers. 'But he's as fat as butter.'

'We like him that way,' said Fleur, tugging the colonel's arm.

'Thanks, Auntie,' said Sebastian. 'And I gather you're about to be swamped in royalties anyway, Valentine, and made into a film?'

'I think I am. I still can't quite believe it.' He laughed. 'But I really think I am. Success after all this time!' Fleur laughed too, not entirely hysterically, and squeezed his arm. He patted her hand.

'Are you all right?' Sebastian asked. 'What's with the cane?'

'Knackered my hip at Reggie's ball. Not sure quite what came over me. Too many painkillers and pirouettes.' He patted Fleur's hand again. 'I was bewitched.'

'I think enchanted's the word,' said Fleur. 'And, now he's really crock, he's been shunted up the queue. The NHS waiting list. We'll be dancing till dawn.'

'In New York.'

'What?'

'We're going to New York,' she said. 'Both of us. And staying in the Carlyle. That lovely boy's arranged everything.'

'Which lovely boy?'

'Shandy's lovely boy.'

'The boy with the silly name. Bright.'

'Silly name, Valentine?' Sebastian put down his plate, wiped his hands on a paper napkin, and pulled two ten-pound notes out of his pocket. 'Ludo, you mean.' He handed them to Valentine. 'Quits. I'm off to the cricket.' He ducked behind Pam's table and pulled out the glass and the flagon of cider. 'I've often thought Pimm's was a little insipid with lemonade. Think I'll give cider a try.'

'We'll join you in a minute,' Fiona said anxiously. 'My godson must be nearing a century.' But he had gone.

With a reek of coal, steam and hot metal, the traction engines edged into the show ring. Reggie stepped out into the enclosure and clapped like mad and we all joined in. There were only two but they were not built for speed, and it took them ten minutes to inch round the ring and collect their prizes. When they had gone, one of the stewards whispered in Reggie's ear.

'Shandy's here,' he said. And there she was, behind Janey's hat.

'I'm sorry about my inappropriate . . . jeans,' she said. 'I was hoping . . .' She held up a small parcel wrapped in brown paper and string. 'Sebastian.'

'He's watching the cricket,' Fiona said, kissing her. 'We're heading that way anyway. Come on.' Pam put a red bag in my hand.

'Fudge to be going on with,' she mouthed. 'For Sebastian.'

'Thanks,' I said. 'I know he loves it.'

'Oh, and what about his beautiful apples? We're clearing away soon.'

'I've got them,' said Shandy, putting an arm round the bottle. 'Safe and sound.'

Fiona's godson was still batting when we arrived, watched by his parents and several friends, including Sebastian, all sitting in deckchairs drinking Pimm's. Sebastian was smoking a cigar and nursing a very dark liquid, in his presentation cup. The flagon of cider, half empty, lay on its side by his chair. Shandy walked up to him, blocking the sun and the match. He put the cigar in his mouth and shaded his eyes, puffing ferociously.

'Excuse me,' he said testily. 'You're in the way.'

'Sebastian,' she said.

'Shandy!' He coughed, wrenching the cigar from his lips and trying to lurch up out of the seat. He rocked forward in an attempt to flip himself up, and again, but with a cigar in one hand and the large glass in the other, he was trapped in the canvas. He lay back and took a deep breath. 'How . . . wonderful.' He placed the glass on the grass, lobbed the cigar under a neighbouring chair and, using both hands this time, tried to bounce upright. 'I thought you were with your guys in New York,' he said, giving up. 'Sorry.'

'You forgot these.' She passed him the pickled apples.

'Thank you,' he said, putting them on the ground.

'This is from me.' She gave him the parcel. He fumbled with the string. 'They still call you the problem, my guys,' she said. He peeled back the paper. 'But of course you're the prize.'

'*Charlotte's Web*,' he said.

'First edition.' She took it from him, opened the cover and gave it back. 'Signed.' He turned the pages gormlessly and two tickets fell out. He held them up.

'Handel's *Messiah* at King's College, Cambridge,' he read.

'After Frinton, I thought, next Saturday?' she said. 'Best beach huts in Essex.'

'Frinton?' This was too much. He threw himself sideways on to the ground, rolled to his knees and scrambled to his feet. 'Perfect,' he said, breathing heavily.

'Good,' she said, and kissed him. He wrapped his arms around her and squeezed and squeezed. She backed off, tottering, and he dragged her into another bear hug, flicking us a V-sign behind her back. When they stopped kissing, she suggested he take her round the show. He noticed the red bag.

'Fudge,' I said, holding it up, 'to be going on with.'

'You have it,' he said, taking Shandy's hand. 'I'm on a diet.'

The Golden Rules

As will be apparent to anyone who has stuck with the book so far, neither Sebastian, Reggie nor I are qualified in any way to give nutritional, dietary or medical advice but, after six months of trying to lose weight, we agreed on a few golden rules that seemed to help us.

Have a Target

Have a target weight and absolute deadline, take it steady and stick to it.

Weigh yourself at the same time of day at least once a week and record your progress. It really does help to see how well you're doing – or badly.

Take it one day at a time and don't be too ambitious. You can keep up a really savage reduction in what you eat for a few days, a few weeks, and maybe even a month or two, but it is simply unsustainable for any length of time – and pretty joyless.

Your weight may fluctuate by several pounds or as much as half a stone each week, but over the long term aim to lose at least one pound a week. This is perfectly feasible – any less and something is wrong. If you eat few enough calories you *will* lose weight.

Go Public But Don't Be a Bore

Don't be a bore about it but admit you're dieting. You can't pretend to be allergic, on antibiotics, or have gastroenteritis for ever.

Try not to be rude or paranoid either. Don't avoid restaurants or refuse invitations because they might not have anything you're 'allowed'. If someone has gone to the trouble of laying on something special, eat it. Feelings are more important than fat fighting.

Do Not Get Hungry

Be ruthless with the contents of your fridge and cupboards. Throw out or lock away everything that could compromise the new regime.

Stock up on what you can eat and drink: cucumbers, olives, carrots, tinned sardines, grapes, hard-boiled eggs, vodka, white wine, etc. If you miss a meal for some reason or can't eat anything somewhere because you feel it would knock you off course, you know you can fill up with the right stuff when you get home. If you can't shoehorn it down, you're not really hungry.

Best to do your own shopping and clearly mark what's yours, in separate packets or boxes if necessary. Getting back after an evening of agonising self-control, sustained purely by the thought of a slab of beef or an apple on your return, only to find it already devoured by a lodger, wife or child can trigger a savage binge reflex, or worse.

Establish what's yours and defend it.

But Eat Less

Of course food can be delicious and the act of eating fun, but small plates force you to take smaller helpings and puny cutlery slows you down.

We feel compelled by conditioning, manners or meanness to clear our plates or empty the bottle. Don't fight your conditioning. Use smaller plates and half-bottles or decanters. Drink half the amount of twice-as-good wine.

Cut It Out

Bite the bullet and give up adding sugar for the duration: you'll get plenty anyway without adding more.

Try to eat and drink fewer fortified or sweet drinks, biscuits, puddings, chocolate, and pretty much everything that tastes sugary. We know what they are. Whatever diet books and their lovely pictures imply, you can't have your cake and eat it. It's amazing how quickly you can do without and how soon old favourites start to taste sickly.

The Soft Option

You do *not* need to give up alcohol, fruit juice or sweet drinks altogether, but they are fattening and you will have to cut down. The fewer calories you drink, the more calories you can eat. There simply may not be a satisfactory alternative to alcoholic drinks, but water really is not *that* bad. The magic number seems to be eight. If you force yourself to have *eight* glasses a day, you'll have less room for other liquids anyway, alcoholic, sugary or not. A glass of water before and during each meal is six glasses already. We often mistake thirst for hunger ... apparently.

Choose Your Battles

Ignore the health angle. You're trying to lose weight, not compete in the Olympics or live for ever – though that may come.

Do not feel obliged to give up booze, fags or salt, or take up exercise, unless feeling exceptionally strong. Exercise makes you fit, not slim. 'Detox' and yoga can wait.

Help Yourself

Get in the zone, psychologically, and stay there. Sticking to the rules seems to help. Find yourself a whopping great carrot and/ or a nasty big stick: more sex? Diabetes? And only do one diet at a time.

Nothing nudges you out of the zone like alcohol. It can make you complacent, silly and rash, stubborn, aggressive and thick. If you are going out for a serious knees-up, lock up, hide or dispose of your carbs and/or calories at home before you leave. To prevent an alcohol-fuelled binge on your return.

Fire up your vanity and shame: put a picture of yourself at your most flabbily unattractive on the fridge door. Eat in front of a mirror, up close, take it off the wall and prop it in front of you. It's surprising how effectively it sours the appetite.

It's fine to skip breakfast, but have lunch before two or you'll crack and end up bingeing on ice cream, carrot cake or whatever else is available.

If you do crack, better overdose on apples than chocolate. All calories and carbs are *not* equal. Better a whole avocado than half an angel cake. Dieting is science but not rocket science. We're greedy, not stupid, but once you feel you've gone too far to salvage the diet for the day, you'll go into Labrador mode and set yourself back a week.

But don't panic. The facts really do seem to suggest that the occasional blow-out fires up the metabolism. Anyway, it's only a diet, and you can always start again. None of us gained more than seven pounds from even an entire day pigging out; lost again in two days. A week of gorging, however, or two or three, is much harder to come back from.

Consolidate

When you reach your target, unless you are very rich, do *not* throw out your old clothes or buy a new suit. Wait. You're not finished. Losing the weight and keeping it lost are entirely different things. You've already ditched the way you lived – or at any rate ate and drank. Now you're going to have to accept some permanent changes ... for six weeks. If you can do it for six weeks, you can do it for twelve. After three months you've cracked it.

What About Us?

Reggie remains a lithe thirteen and a half stone on the Fast Diet, but only by fasting for three, not two days a week.

I try to avoid carbs, going back on the Atkins proper for a while when I gain more than five pounds: surprisingly often.

Sebastian is . . . doing his research.